know your chances

know your chances

Understanding Health Statistics

Steven Woloshin, MD, MS, Lisa M. Schwartz, MD, MS,
and H. Gilbert Welch, MD, MPH

UNIVERSITY OF CALIFORNIA PRESS

Berkeley Los Angeles London

University of California Press, one of the most distinguished university presses in the United States, enriches lives around the world by advancing scholarship in the humanities, social sciences, and natural sciences. Its activities are supported by the UC Press Foundation and by philanthropic contributions from individuals and institutions. For more information, visit www.ucpress.edu.

University of California Press
Berkeley and Los Angeles, California

University of California Press, Ltd.
London, England

Photo credits: p. ii, luoman/istock.com; p. 9, PeskyMonkey/istock.com; p. 35, superseker/istock.com; p. 65, jubrancoelho/istock.com; p. 85, Razvan/istock.com; p. 115, RapidEye/istock.com.

Library of Congress Cataloging-in-Publication Data

Woloshin, Steven
   Know your chances : understanding health statistics / Steven Woloshin, Lisa M. Schwartz, H. Gilbert Welch.
      p.   cm.
   Includes bibliographical references and index.
   ISBN 978-0-520-25222-6 (pbk. : alk. paper)
   1. Health risk assessment—Popular works.   2. Medical statistics—Popular works.   I. Schwartz, Lisa M.   II. Welch, H. Gilbert.   III. Title.
   RA427.3.W65   2008
   614.4'2—dc22   2008026119

Manufactured in the United States of America

17   16   15   14   13   12   11   10   09   08
10   9   8   7   6   5   4   3   2   1

The paper used in this publication meets the minimum requirements of ANSI / NISO Z39.48–1992 (R 1997) *(Permanence of Paper)*.

The publisher gratefully acknowledges the generous support of James and Carlin Naify as members of the Publisher's Circle of the University of California Press Foundation.

We would like to thank the Department of Veterans Affairs,

the National Cancer Institute, and the Robert Wood Johnson

Foundation's Generalist Faculty Scholar Program for their support.

And we thank Emma, Eli, and Heather for making everything

so much fun. This book is dedicated to the memory of Leonard

Schwartz.

Numbers can make people sick.

But they don't have to.

Learn how to make them help you.

CONTENTS

what this book is about

Every day we are faced with news stories, ads, and public service announcements that describe health threats and suggest ways we can protect ourselves. It's impossible to watch television, open a magazine, read a newspaper, or go online without being bombarded by messages about the dangers we face.

Many of the messages are intended to be scary, warning us that we are surrounded by danger and hinting that everything we do or neglect to do brings us one step closer to cancer, heart disease, and death. Other messages are intended to be full of hope, reassuring us that technological miracles and breakthrough drugs can save us all. And many messages do both: they use fear to make us feel vulnerable and then provide some hope by telling us what we can do (or buy) to lower our risk. In addition, as you may suspect, a great many of these messages are wildly exaggerated: many of the risks we hear about are really not so big, and the benefits of many of the miraculous breakthroughs are often pretty small.

As a result, we are often left misinformed and confused. But it doesn't have to be that way.

The goal of this book is to help you better understand health information by teaching you about the numbers behind the messages—the medical statistics on which the claims are based. The book will also familiarize you with risk charts, which are designed to help you put your health concerns in perspective. By learning to understand the numbers and knowing what questions to ask, you'll be able to see through the hype and find the credible information—if any—that remains.

Don't worry: this is not a math book (only a few simple calculations are required). Instead, this is a book that will teach you what numbers to look for in health messages and how to tell when the medical statistics don't support the message. This book will help you develop the basic skills you need to become a better consumer of health messages, and these skills will foster better communication between you and your doctor.

Confusing Health Messages

Unfortunately, it can be hard to make sense of health messages. It can be difficult to figure out just how big the threats are or how well the drugs, tests, or behaviors highlighted in the messages actually work.

Why is it so hard? First, there are problems with the messages: many are incomplete, misleading, or overstated. It's easy to understand why. The message writers may not know what they're doing—or, more likely, they may know exactly what they're doing. Without doubt, the media, medical journals, pharmaceutical companies, researchers, research funders, and academic institutions all have an interest in being associated with work that is perceived to be big, new, and important. That is a recipe for exaggeration.

Second, there are problems with the audiences who receive the messages. Most people haven't been taught how to "read" health messages critically—in other words, they don't know which numbers to look for, how to recognize when key data are missing, how to put messages in perspective, or how to think about the evidence behind the messages and assess what counts as credible evidence.

This book will teach you how to look at health messages critically and how to understand the statistics behind them. We want to help you develop a healthy skepticism that, as illustrated here, will let you push back against

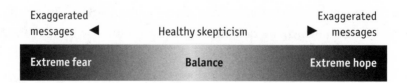

unfounded, exaggerated claims. We are not saying that there's never anything to fear or that there's no reason for hope. We are saying that it takes some effort and skill to see through exaggeration and to recognize real dangers and benefits.

A Quick Word on Words

Before we go further and start looking at health messages, we want to ensure that we're being clear about some basic language.

Risk: To most people, the word *risk* means "danger": for example, "lion taming is a high-risk hobby." But *risk* is also used to mean the *chance* that something will happen to you: for example, "in this group of patients, the risk of heart attack is about 10 percent." In this book, we use *risk* as a synonym for *chance*. Usually, we'll be talking about the chance of something bad happening (like having a heart attack). Strictly speaking, risk can refer to the chance of anything—good or bad—happening. This leads us to the next key word, *outcome*.

Outcome: The *outcome* is the "something" that may happen—maybe death or maybe a medical event such as a heart attack or a cancer diagnosis. Thus, risk is the chance that you will experience some outcome. For example, a man may be interested to know his risk of prostate cancer. That is, he wants to know the chance of something occurring. The "something" here—the outcome—is getting prostate cancer.

Statistics: The last word we want to introduce is one that may strike fear into the hearts of many readers: *statistics*. Statistics are just numbers that summarize information. They are based on observations of large groups of people and are useful in predicting what is likely to happen in the future. The statistics we focus on summarize the chance that an outcome will happen. These *risk statistics* are simply fractions. The numerator (the top number in the fraction) is the number of people who actually experience the outcome. The denominator (the bottom number) is the number of people who could potentially experience it. For example, if 10 lion tamers get bitten among the 100 lion tamers that we observe for a year, the fraction looks like this: 10 / 100. That is, a lion tamer's risk of being bitten is 10 out of 100, or 10 percent per year. The risk statistic here summarizes the chance that a lion tamer will experience the unpleasant outcome of getting chomped on by a lion.

Statistics can be complex and tricky—but they don't have to be. And as this book will show you, good statistics usually aren't.

An Overview of What Comes Next

This book is intended for anyone who encounters health messages—in other words, for everyone. We don't aim to turn you into doctors or statisticians; rather, the goal is to help you make sense of the messages. Because many people are intimidated by statistics, we worked hard to make the book non-threatening and engaging, by including plenty of illustrations, walking you through examples, and offering the more technical explanations in separate sections.

The book is divided into four basic parts, with a final section that provides extra help.

Part One: What Is My Risk?

The first chapter focuses on how to analyze messages about risk—specifically, how to find the fundamental information needed to give the message meaning, and how to do one or two simple, relevant calculations. You'll learn to ask the following questions: "Risk of what? How big is the risk? Does the risk information reasonably apply to me?" We'll also look at how messages are framed: subtle changes in how risk messages are presented can make a big difference in how people interpret—and act on—identical information.

Chapter 2 highlights a key issue: people are typically given risk information in isolation, with no idea of how a particular risk compares to other important health risks. This chapter stresses the importance of perspective in interpreting risk messages. To illustrate perspective, we introduce risk charts, simple tables that show a person's chance of dying over a 10-year period from various causes (for instance, heart attack, stroke, pneumonia, flu, accidents, or cancer) and from all causes combined.

Chapter 3 explains how to use the risk charts and reinforces the importance of perspective in interpreting risk information. Specifically, we focus on how basic characteristics such as age, gender, and smoking greatly influence many risks. We'll present two risk charts—one for men and one for women—that indicate the chance of death for people who have never smoked and people who currently smoke. By comparing risks of death from various causes, and all causes combined, you can get some perspective on the relative importance of these risks at different ages. Also, by comparing the current smoker and nonsmoker risks, you'll understand why all doctors agree that not smoking is the single most important thing you can do to prolong life.

Part Two: Can I Reduce My Risk?

Just as chapter 1 teaches you how to understand risk messages, chapter 4 teaches you how to understand messages about risk reduction. You'll learn to ask these key questions: "What outcome is being reduced? And how big is the reduction?"

Chapter 4 also builds on the idea of figuring out just how well the information in a health message applies to you. Like messages about risk, messages about risk reduction are most relevant if they are based on studies of people *like you*. This chapter emphasizes a key point: the size of the risk reduction you can expect from an intervention depends on your starting risk—in other words, the higher your risk to begin with, the more you stand to benefit from an intervention.

Understanding the benefit means understanding the importance of different outcomes—the way in which benefit is measured. Chapter 5 introduces you to the *pyramid of benefit*, which can help you assess the value of interventions, ranging from the least important interventions, which improve only things that you don't directly experience (such as blood test results) to interventions that change how you feel or how long you live.

Part Three: Does Risk Reduction Have Downsides?

Treatments always have downsides: cost, inconvenience, bothersome side effects, or, rarely, major life-threatening consequences. Chapter 6 teaches you how to think about side effects in order to decide whether the health interventions you hear about are worth considering.

Chapter 7 provides practical advice on how to put the lessons of the previous chapters into action: how to weigh the benefits and downsides of treatments. This means determining how large the risk reduction can be and what you have to do to achieve it. Treatments that have a lot of downsides are worth doing only if they have a lot of benefit.

Part Four: Developing a Healthy Skepticism

As we said before, the health messages you encounter every day in the media are often misleading and overstated. Chapter 8 reviews the strategies that the authors of these messages sometimes use to exaggerate the importance of risk (or risk reduction) and provides some guidance on how to be a healthy skeptic. We also take a look at some of the most commonly misused (and exaggerated) statistics around: *survival statistics*. These numbers tell you what percentage of people are still alive at a specified time after a diagnosis (typically, you hear about 5-year or 10-year survival). Although survival statistics can be very important when they are used correctly, these seemingly simple numbers are easily misused and can cause lots of confusion. By the end of chapter 8, you'll know how these statistics work and how to tell when they are being abused.

Chapter 9 reminds you that getting the numbers is not the whole story. You must still decide whether or not to believe them. We offer some guidance about how to judge the believability of research findings and a set of cautions to keep in mind when you hear about different kinds of research (for instance, observational studies or randomized trials). The chapter ends with a caution about interpreting preliminary findings, such as research presented at meetings of medical or scientific associations. Because such preliminary findings are not the final results, the conclusions of the study may change (a lot) over time as the study matures.

In chapter 10, we urge you to think about who is behind the numbers you hear in health messages. Some of the sources of the information you encounter have important interests besides your health. Unfortunately, these other interests may tempt the people behind the numbers to distort or to spin the information to make their message look more compelling—for example, by maximizing the apparent benefit or by minimizing the potential harm of interventions. Many conflicts of interest are financial, but some are nonfinancial: scientists and physicians may benefit professionally by being associated with work that appears to be groundbreaking, new, or important. When you evaluate the credibility of the scientists and the research behind a health message, it's worth asking whether any of these conflicts exist.

Extra Help

Finally, the Extra Help section provides tools that you can use to make sense of health messages in the future. It includes a quick summary of the entire book, a glossary of key terms, a number converter that helps you rewrite numbers into an easy-to-understand format, and the full version of the risk charts discussed earlier in the book. We have also provided a list of credible sources for health statistics and a section of notes with references for some of the material we present.

How to Use This Book

Much of the information in this book may be new to you. That's okay. It's new to lots of people—including many doctors. But we're confident that almost everyone can learn to make better sense of the health statistics that we see in real life. To help you along, we have included the following features:

Quizzes are meant for everybody. Do them before you look at the answers. Quizzes will help you know how well you've understood the material—and help build your confidence. We urge you to do them and not to proceed until you understand the right answer, since what comes next often builds on what came before.

Learn More boxes are meant for readers who want to investigate topics a little more deeply. You can safely skip these boxes and still get the big picture, but we think you'll learn more if you take the extra time to read them.

We have tried to make this book short and simple. But there is still a lot here. You'll do best if you take time to digest and reflect on what you learn. Try reading the book in a few sittings, and take some intermissions. Good luck!

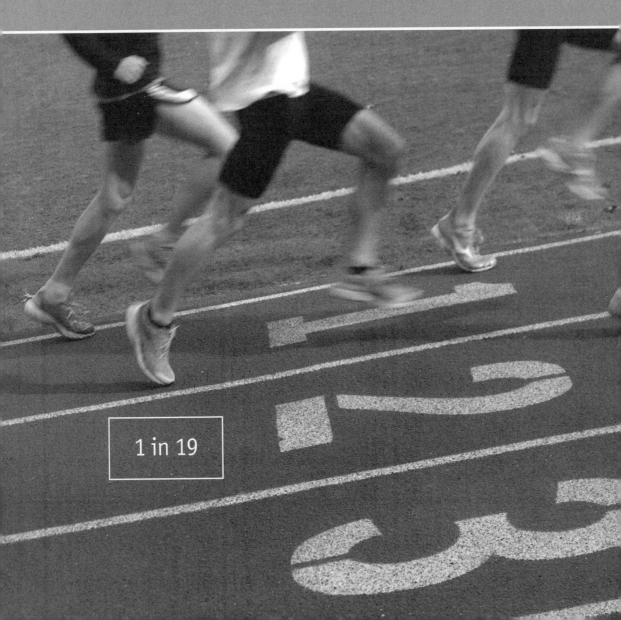

what is my risk?

1 in 19

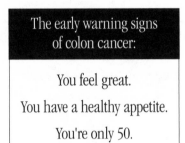

The early warning signs
of colon cancer:

You feel great.
You have a healthy appetite.
You're only 50.

For many people, this is a pretty scary message. It says that you need to worry: if you feel well, you may have colon cancer (cancer of the large intestine or rectum). The purpose of the message, which ran in the *New York Times* as part of an advertisement for the Memorial Sloan-Kettering Cancer Center, is to motivate people to go in for colon cancer screening. But some key information is missing from this message. For starters, it doesn't tell you how likely colon cancer is. If your chance of getting colon cancer is large, there is more reason to worry than if your chance is small. This information might help you decide whether to try to lower your risk.

Do all 50-year-old people who feel great and have healthy appetites really have colon cancer? **QUIZ**

    a. Yes
    b. No

The correct answer is no, of course not. The vast majority do not have colon cancer. Do you know how common colon cancer is? It turns out that most people—including many doctors—don't have a good understanding of how common different diseases really are. Messages like the Sloan-Kettering ad are good at catching people's attention. Unfortunately, they can leave you with either an exaggerated sense of risk or a feeling of confusion. In the next few pages, we'll try to help you understand how big your risk of colon cancer really is.

One word of warning: all the numbers we'll show you are real. Most are U.S. government health statistics. The numbers may seem hard to believe because they will seem to change a lot as you go through the chapter. But that's part of our point: we'll be saying the same thing in different ways. And, as you'll see, how you say things matters. Seeing different ways of expressing numbers will help you understand what the numbers mean.

Consider this message:

> "Colon cancer will strike about 150,000 Americans."

This statement illustrates a common strategy used to highlight—really, to exaggerate—risk. The message uses an attention-grabbing large number, but it lacks any information that would allow you to put the number in context. To understand what the number means, you need to know more.

To make sense of this message, you need to ask, "150,000 out of how many?"—that is, how many people could possibly get colon cancer? (Scientists refer to this group as the *population at risk*.) In the United States, the number of people who could develop colon cancer is the entire American population, about 300 million people. So we can say that colon cancer strikes 150,000 out of these 300 million (300,000,000). The number 150,000 divided by 300,000,000 is 0.0005—or 5 out of 10,000. Some people like to give these numbers as percentages; in this case, the number would be 0.05 percent. (See the Learn More box on page 13.)

Highlighting the number of cancer cases (or occurrences of any disease) without mentioning the number of people at risk is a common way to make

Learn More

Calculating Risk

Risk can be expressed as a fraction. The numerator is the number of people who actually experience the outcome, and the denominator is the number of people who could possibly experience it (sometimes called the population at risk). For example, consider the risk of getting colon cancer:

$$\text{Risk} = \frac{\text{number of people diagnosed with colon cancer (numerator)}}{\text{number of people at risk (denominator)}}$$

$$= \frac{150{,}000 \text{ Americans diagnosed}}{300{,}000{,}000 \text{ Americans}}$$

$$= \frac{5}{10{,}000} = 0.0005$$

So, here, the risk of getting colon cancer is 0.0005.

Many people find numbers like this—with all those zeros after the decimal point—hard to understand. In this case, the number means that, on average, a person's chance of getting colon cancer is five ten-thousandths (0.0005). There are many ways to describe the 0.0005 risk of colon cancer. For example, all the different expressions shown in this table say exactly the same thing:

Format Goal	Decimal Format	Multiplication Needed		"Out of How Many?" Format
Risk per 1 person	0.0005	× 1	=	0.0005 out of 1 person
Risk per 10 people	0.0005	× 10	=	0.005 out of 10 people
Risk per 100 people	0.0005	× 100	=	0.05 out of 100 people
Risk per 1,000 people	0.0005	× 1,000	=	0.5 out of 1,000 people
Risk per 10,000 people	0.0005	× 10,000	=	5 out of 10,000 people
Risk per 100,000 people	0.0005	× 100,000	=	50 out of 100,000 people

Risk per 100 people is often expressed as a percentage. "Percent" is just a fancy way of saying "out of 100." So you can say "0.05 percent" instead of "0.05 per 100 people"; both expressions mean the same thing.

Scientists tend to favor the expression that lets them use whole numbers rather than decimals—in this case, they would say "5 out of 10,000."

risks sound big. Your attention is focused on the large number (for example, 150,000) instead of the small percentage (0.05 percent). Therefore, when you hear about the number of people with a disease, you should always ask, "Out of how many?"

QUIZ Cervical cancer will strike about 13,000 women in the United States.

What information is missing?

    a. Total number of American women

    b. Total number of Americans

The correct answer is a, the total number of American women. That answers the question "13,000 out of how many?" This quiz contained a trick question (sorry). It required you to know that only women can get cervical cancer. Why? Because only women have a cervix (it's the opening to the uterus, or womb). But this trick question illustrates an important point. To really understand a risk, you need to know two things: how many people experience the outcome (here, the 13,000 women whom cervical cancer strikes), and how many people could experience the outcome (here, the total number of women, which is about 150 million). So a woman's risk of cervical cancer is 13,000 divided by 150,000,000 women, which is 0.00009, or 0.009 percent.

The cervical cancer example demonstrates an important point: the population at risk (the "out of how many?" part of the risk calculation) refers only to people who could possibly experience the outcome. Since only women can get cervical cancer, it would be wrong (and would make no sense) to include men when calculating the risk. The same would be true of ovarian cancer, since men don't have ovaries. Similarly, because men have a prostate (a gland right below the bladder that helps produce semen) and women do not, only men can get prostate cancer, so women are excluded from the population at risk for prostate cancer.

But even when both sexes can experience the outcome, looking at risk separately for men and for women can be useful. When the chances of the outcome differ substantially by sex, it is of little value to calculate a single risk for the combined group. For example, both men and women can get breast cancer (both have breast tissue), but the disease is at least 100 times more common in women because women's breasts are much more hormonally active. That is why breast cancer risk is calculated separately for men and for women.

Remember, when you hear about a risk, be clear about how many people actually experience the outcome and how many people could *possibly* experience the outcome.

Here's another way you may have heard people talk about colon cancer risk:

> "Colon cancer will strike 1 in 19 people."

Whoa! What happened? This statistic certainly sounds very different from 5 out of 10,000. (Don't worry—we'll explain why soon.)

Many people find statistics like 1 in 19 confusing (we call an expression like this the "1 in ___" format). Because we don't usually come across things in groups of 19, it isn't surprising that we have trouble imagining what 1 in 19 means (or 1 in 13, or 1 in 97, or any unusual group, for that matter). The other problem with numbers like 1 in 19 comes up when we try to compare two such statistics: unless the group sizes (the "in 19" parts) are exactly the same, it's really hard to make comparisons. Try the following quiz to see what we mean:

QUIZ

The chance of bladder cancer is 1 in 43.

Which is greater, the chance of bladder cancer (1 in 43) or the chance of colon cancer (1 in 19)?

    a. Bladder cancer
    b. Colon cancer

The correct answer is b, colon cancer. When people compare numbers like 1 in 43 and 1 in 19, it's easy to get confused because the larger chance (in this case, the chance of colon cancer) is "out of" a smaller number. If you got the wrong answer to this quiz or felt unsure, you might find it easier to understand with pictures.

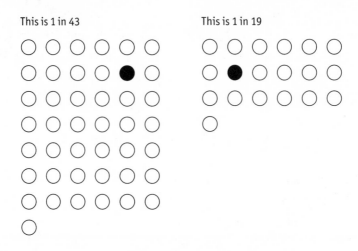

This is 1 in 43   This is 1 in 19

But this can get kind of awkward. Consider breast cancer among men. The chance is about 1 in 909. Who wants to draw that? (Don't you have something better to do?)

To make comparisons easier, it helps to use the same number of people every time. This is usually done by comparing the number of people "out of 100" or "out of 1,000." In this book, we will use "out of 1,000" (because many health risks are smaller than 1 in 100). The easiest way to get the numbers into the "out of 1,000" format is to divide them. (See the Learn More box on page 17.) Here, we have converted the numbers from the quiz:

$$\text{Bladder cancer risk} = \frac{1}{43} = 0.023 = 23 \text{ out of } 1,000$$

$$\text{Colon cancer risk} = \frac{1}{19} = 0.053 = 53 \text{ out of } 1,000$$

Now it's easy to see that colon cancer is the larger risk. (Don't worry about the changing numbers you're seeing for colon cancer risk; we'll soon explain what's going on.)

Clearly, how you say things matters: some ways are just easier to understand than others. That's why we included the number converter in the Extra Help section of this book (see pages 126–127). Here's an excerpt from the number converter, in which each row shows four different ways of saying the same thing. You can also use the number converter to make estimates: for example, 1 in 19 would be between 1 in 10 and 1 in 20 but much closer to 1 in 20.

1 in ____	Decimal	Percent	____ out of 1,000
1 in 10	0.10	10%	100 out of 1,000
1 in 20	0.05	5%	50 out of 1,000
1 in 25	0.04	4%	40 out of 1,000

Now let's put the two colon cancer risk messages together:

"Colon cancer will strike 53 out of 1,000 people."

"Colon cancer will strike 5 out of 10,000 people."

How can both of these statements be true? The first statistic, 53 out of 1,000, is the chance of colon cancer over a *lifetime*. The statistic means that, on average, colon cancer strikes 53 out of 1,000 people (which is the same as 530 out of 10,000) at some point between birth and death. The number we introduced early in the chapter—5 out of 10,000—is the chance of colon cancer over the course of *1 year*. As you can see, the period of time under consideration matters a lot. Your chance of cancer increases over time. The longer the time, the larger the chance.

You can think of it like the chance of catching a cold. Let's say that you're feeling fine right now. The chance that you'll catch a cold in the next few minutes is extremely small. The chance that you'll catch a cold in the next few days is also very small. But, over time, the chance increases. Most people would agree that the chance that they'll catch a cold in the next 10 years is close to certain. So the longer the time period, the bigger the risk. Unless you know the time frame (such as 1 year, 10 years, or a lifetime), it's very hard to know what a risk statistic means.

Which of these time frames is right? Many organizations, including the American Cancer Society, prefer to present lifetime cancer risks. Such life-time risks, which are based on long time periods (the average person born nowadays in the United States will live about 78 years), often seem impres-sive. If a person lives to an old age, it means more time for a cancer (or any other outcome) to occur. So presenting lifetime risks tends to make the risks look big. On the other hand, presenting risks for a short time period, like a single year, tends to make the risks look pretty small. (Perhaps too small, because most risks accumulate over time.)

Many people are more interested in their chance of cancer in the foresee-able future than in the more abstract time frame of an entire lifetime. For that reason, we'll usually talk about the chance over the next 10 years. The 10-year time frame is arbitrary, but it makes sense to us. It's not too long (so it's easy to imagine), and it's not too short (so the risks aren't forced to look too small). And it allows time to do things like change your lifestyle to reduce your risk. (More on that later.)

To summarize how much the time matters, here are risk statistics for all three time frames. On average, colon cancer will strike . . .

5 out of 10,000 people in 1 year
5 out of 1,000 people in 10 years
53 out of 1,000 people in a lifetime

These numbers might seem to imply that the average person lives more than 100 years (because you would have to multiply the 10-year risk by more than 10 to get the lifetime risk). But the lifetime risk is higher than you might expect because the risk of cancer (in general) increases exponentially as you get older. In the case of colon cancer, the risk is extremely low in people younger than 40 and starts going up faster and faster around age 60.

It's clear that the time frame matters—a lot! If someone tells you that colon cancer will strike 53 out of 1,000 people (or any number for that matter), you need to ask, "Over how long a time?"

Here's the revised colon cancer message, which now includes the time frame:

"Over the next 10 years, colon cancer will strike 5 out of 1,000 people."

The message is becoming clearer, but some important information is still missing. What does the word *strike* mean? Does it mean *getting* colon cancer, or does it mean *dying* from colon cancer? Of course, these are not the same. Not all people with colon cancer die from it. To make sense of this message, you need to ask, "Risk of what? The risk of getting a disease or the risk of dying from it?"

For most diseases, getting the disease is much more likely than dying from it. Although many people believe that cancer is a death sentence, fortunately that is far from the case. By comparing your chance of getting cancer to your chance of dying from that cancer, you can get a sense of how deadly the cancer really is.

Guess the chance of dying from colon cancer in the next 10 years:

> a. 103 out of 1,000
> b. 53 out of 1,000
> c. 5 out of 1,000
> d. 2 out of 1,000

The correct answer is d, 2 out of 1,000. That is, out of 1,000 people, we estimate that 5 will get colon cancer and 2 will die of colon cancer over the next 10 years. (Note that, logically, the chance of dying from colon cancer must be lower than—or equal to—the chance of getting it, so the answer could not have been more than 5.)

QUIZ Compare the following messages about 10-year risks:

> Jones's chance of dying of colon cancer is 2 out of 1,000.
> Smith's chance of *not* dying of colon cancer is 998 out of 1,000.

Who is more likely to die of colon cancer in the next 10 years?

> a. Jones
> b. Smith
> c. They have the same chance
> d. Can't tell from the information given

The correct answer is c—they have the same chance. If the two statements about Jones and Smith don't sound the same to you, don't worry; most people react differently to these two sets of numbers. A 2 out of 1,000 chance of dying from colon cancer sounds scarier than a 998 out of 1,000 chance of not dying from colon cancer, even though these two statements say exactly the same thing. It's a bit like an optical illusion—a small change in perspective makes a big difference in what you see.

> 2 out of 1,000 die = 998 out of 1,000 live

How you are given information—being told that the glass is half-empty rather than half-full—can really affect how you feel about it (even though the amount of water is the same). Presenting the same information in different ways is called *framing*. There is no reason to think that one way of framing a risk ("2 out of 1,000 die") is more correct than another ("998 out of 1,000 do not die"). The important thing is to be aware of the influence of framing and to try and get past it—in other words, to be sure that it doesn't cloud your objectivity.

One way to do this—to decide how you really feel about a risk—is to give yourself a chance to react to both versions of a risk message. When you hear a risk presented one way (such as the chance of dying), rewrite it the other way (the chance of not dying), so that you can look at it in both frames. Fortunately, you don't need to do this all the time—it could get pretty tedious—but it's a good idea to try recasting risk messages once in a while, especially when you find yourself surprised by a message about a seemingly big risk.

For example, using the colon cancer example, you could say:

> "Over 10 years, the average person's chance of dying from colon cancer is 2 out of 1,000. Another way of saying this is that their chance of *not* dying from colon cancer is 998 out of 1,000."

This statement is pretty complete: it is clear about what outcome is under discussion, how big the risk is, and how long the time frame is. Plus it lets you see that the half-empty glass is also in fact half-full.

But there's still a problem. This complete statement may be quite useful to the average person. But what about you? Let's say you are 65 years old, and the average person is 36 years old. Do you think that your chance of getting colon cancer is the same as the average person's? It's always important to ask, "Whose risk are we talking about?" You are not necessarily the "average person."

Since everyone's risk is different, statistics about risk are most helpful when they are based on people like you. What does it mean, to be "like you"? Well, in health statistics, age and sex are generally the most important predictors of what will happen to you. So the most relevant health numbers for you are ones about people who are of your age and sex. Helping you learn how to put risk into perspective by considering age and sex and by comparing risk across various diseases is what the next chapter is all about.

putting risk in perspective **2**

Look at the circles in the middle of these two illustrations. The one on the left is bigger, isn't it?

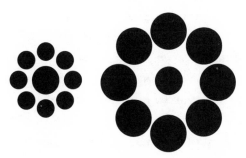

No. The circles in the middle are exactly the same size. The one on the left looks bigger, but this is just an optical illusion. The small circles in the lefthand picture make the middle circle look relatively big, while the big circles in the righthand picture make the middle circle look relatively small. The point is that people do not interpret information in isolation.

Even when news stories, ads, or public service announcements do a good job of providing risk statistics (that is, including the number of people who experience the outcome, the number who could experience it, and the time frame), you still need more information to make the numbers meaningful. The numbers need to be put in perspective. One kind of perspective, described in the previous chapter, lets you compare your chance of getting a disease with your chance of dying from it. This sort of perspective helps you appreciate how dangerous the disease is—and, for many people, knowing their chance of dying from a disease is really the most important information.

For much of this book, we focus on the chance of dying. In this chapter, we provide ways to get perspective on this chance. We'll start by taking age and sex into account to help you see how a risk applies to you as an individual. Finally, we'll add another kind of perspective: how one disease compares to others.

In this chapter and the next, we'll introduce you to the "risk charts" that provide this perspective. These charts show the chance that people of different ages will die from various causes. We created these charts using data from the federal government's vital statistics records—the best available data.

About 5 years ago, we published the charts and our method for calculating them in the *Journal of the National Cancer Institute*.[1] Since then, we have updated the charts using the most recent data available (which is from 2004) and refined our calculations. The new charts have just been published in a recent issue of the *Journal of the National Cancer Institute*.[2]

We'll start with a small excerpt of the chart showing the chance that women of different ages will die from colon cancer in the next 10 years. To use the chart, begin with the first column and find the age you're interested in. Then look in the next column to see the number of colon cancer deaths that will occur among 1,000 women that age in the next 10 years.

The numbers in the chart tell you how many out of 1,000 women of various ages will die in the next 10 years from colon cancer.

Age (Years)	Colon Cancer Deaths
45	1
50	1
55	2
60	3
65	5
70	7
75	10

To be sure you understand how to use the chart, please answer the following question:

What is the chance that a 50-year-old woman will die of colon cancer in the next **QUIZ** 10 years?

    a. 5 out of 1,000
    b. 2 out of 1,000
    c. 1 out of 1,000

If you've read the chart correctly, you'll see that the answer is c, 1 out of 1,000. We'll be using this kind of chart a lot, so it's important that you understand how to read it.

As you can see, this risk increases with age. For example, by age 75, a woman's chance of dying from colon cancer in the next 10 years is 10 out of 1,000.

A Broader Perspective

A 50-year-old woman has a 1 out of 1,000 chance of dying from colon cancer in the next 10 years. Is that a large or small chance? To decide, it helps to compare this risk with other risks. Comparing the risk of dying from different diseases helps you appreciate which are the biggest threats you face (the ones you might want to do something about) and which threats are less worrisome.

The next chart compares a woman's risk of dying from colon cancer to her risk of dying from other causes. For simplicity, we show only the information for 50-year-old women.

The numbers in the chart tell you how many out of 1,000 fifty-year-old women will die in the next 10 years from . . .

| Age | Vascular Disease | | Cancer | | | | | Infection | | | Lung Disease | Accidents |
	Heart Attack	Stroke	Lung	Breast	Colon	Ovarian	Cervical	Pneumonia	Flu	AIDS	COPD	
50	4	1	1	4	1	1						2

Note: Shaded portions mean that the chance is less than 1 out of 1,000. COPD is chronic obstructive pulmonary disease, which includes emphysema and chronic bronchitis.

Let's make sure you understand how to use the chart:

QUIZ Mrs. Jones is a 50-year-old woman. Which is the bigger risk for Mrs. Jones?

  a. Colon cancer
  b. Heart attack

The correct answer is b, heart attack. The chart shows that a 50-year-old woman's chance of dying from a heart attack in the next 10 years is 4 out of 1,000, while her chance of dying from colon cancer during that time is 1 out of 1,000. Her chance of dying from colon cancer is about the same as her chance of dying from stroke or ovarian cancer but is higher than her chance of dying from cervical cancer, pneumonia, or AIDS.

QUIZ Mrs. Jones is a 50-year-old woman. What is her chance of dying from all causes combined in the next 10 years?

  a. 1 out of 1,000
  b. 8 out of 1,000
  c. 14 out of 1,000
  d. More than 14 out of 1,000

The correct answer is d, more than 14 out of 1,000. Sorry—this may have seemed like another trick question. Of course, the chance of dying from all causes combined is greater than the chance of dying from colon cancer.

To get the correct answer, however, you had to realize that there are many other causes of death besides the ones included in the charts (for example, homicide, suicide, other cancers—such as stomach cancer, bone cancer, or melanoma—kidney failure, infections, and so on). So the number had to be greater than 14, which is the sum of the numbers listed in the chart. The actual answer is 37 out of 1,000.

Knowing the chance of dying from all causes combined adds another important perspective: it allows you to see how each individual cause of death contributes to this total. Because there are so many causes of death, you can't simply add up the numbers in the row. So we now add a final column on the righthand side of the chart: the chance of dying from all causes combined.

The numbers in the chart tell you how many out of 1,000 fifty-year-old women will die in the next 10 years from . . .

Age	Vascular Disease		Cancer					Infection			Lung Disease	Accidents	All Causes Combined
	Heart Attack	Stroke	Lung	Breast	Colon	Ovarian	Cervical	Pneumonia	Flu	AIDS	COPD		
50	4	1	1	4	1	1						2	37

Note: Shaded portions mean that the chance is less than 1 out of 1,000. COPD is chronic obstructive pulmonary disease, which includes emphysema and chronic bronchitis.

To decide how you really feel about a risk message, remember to give yourself an opportunity to react to both the "glass half-empty" and "glass half-full" versions. In the previous chapter, we mentioned framing, the idea that alternate ways of presenting the same information can elicit very different feelings. We suggested that when you hear a risk reported as the chance of dying, you might try reframing it as the chance of not dying. We have done just that in the following charts. Each chart indicates what is likely to happen to 1,000 fifty-year-old women over the next 10 years.

Age	Vascular Disease		Cancer					Infection			Lung Disease	Accidents	All Causes Combined
	Heart Attack	Stroke	Lung	Breast	Colon	Ovarian	Cervical	Pneumonia	Flu	AIDS	COPD		
50	4	1	1	4	1	1	<1	<1	<1	<1	<1	2	37

B: *The chance of* not dying *in the next 10 years*

Age	Vascular Disease		Cancer					Infection			Lung Disease	Accidents	All Causes Combined
	Heart Attack	Stroke	Lung	Breast	Colon	Ovarian	Cervical	Pneumonia	Flu	AIDS	COPD		
50	996	999	999	996	999	999	>999	>999	>999	>999	>999	998	963

Remember, to understand risk, you need to know the outcome being considered, the size of the risk, and the time frame. And it's important to be aware of how the risk is presented (the framing). But in addition you need perspective: a way to compare this risk with others. Comparing makes it possible for you to decide how big or important a risk really is. Perspective really matters. But don't just take our word for it:

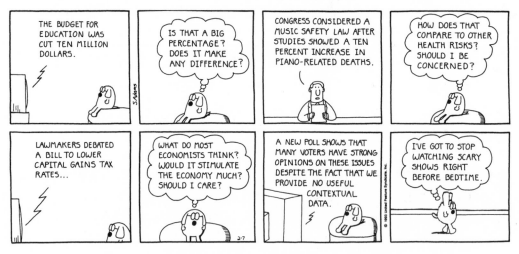

DILBERT © Scott Adams / Dist. by United Feature Syndicate, Inc.

risk charts: a way to get perspective 3

How does a specific risk compare to other risks for your age group and your gender? Answering this question is precisely the purpose of our risk charts. Because the risk charts are so important to understanding risk and providing perspective, we want you to take a close look at them. (The full charts appear in the Extra Help section at the end of the book, pages 128–129.)

We created two risk charts: one for men and one for women. The columns in the charts indicate various causes of death. Each chart shows the 10-year chance of dying from these causes for people of different ages. There are two rows of numbers for each age: the rows in regular type are for people who have never smoked (individuals who don't smoke now and who have smoked fewer than 100 cigarettes in their lifetime, referred to in the charts as "never smoked"), and the rows in **bold** type are for people who currently smoke (individuals who have smoked at least 100 cigarettes and who smoke now).

Why do we give separate numbers for current smokers and people who never smoked? It's because smoking has such a strong influence on your risk of dying. You probably know that smoking causes lung cancer. But smoking also makes a big difference when we look at many other diseases, such as heart attack, stroke, and pneumonia.

To highlight how much smoking matters, let's take a look at part of the chart for women.

Find the line with a specific age and smoking status. The numbers in that row tell you how many out of 1,000 women in that group will die in the next 10 years from . . .

Age	Smoking Status	Vascular Disease		Cancer					Infection			Lung Disease	Accidents	All Causes Combined
		Heart Attack	Stroke	Lung	Breast	Colon	Ovarian	Cervical	Pneumonia	Flu	AIDS	COPD		
50	Never smoked	4	1	1	4	1	1						2	37
	Smoker	13	5	14	4	1	1		1			4	2	69
55	Never smoked	8	2	2	6	2	2	1	1			1	2	55
	Smoker	20	6	26	5	2	2	1	1			9	2	110

Note: Shaded portions mean that the chance is less than 1 out of 1,000. COPD is chronic obstructive pulmonary disease, which includes emphysema and chronic bronchitis.

In the chart, find the rows for 50-year-old women. For women who never smoked, the chance of dying in the next 10 years from all causes combined is 37 out of 1,000. (Note that this is the same row of data we used in chapter 2.) For current smokers, the corresponding risk is almost twice as high: 69 out of 1,000.

What about former smokers? Things are a little more complicated for them. That's because risks for smoking-related diseases drop after you quit smoking. But it's hard to say how much the risks drop. Your change in risk depends mostly on two basic factors: how much you smoked (when you started and how many cigarettes you smoked each day), and how long it's been since you quit. If you are a former smoker, you can also use the risk charts: your risk falls somewhere between that of current smokers and people who never smoked. The longer it's been since you smoked and the less you smoked, the closer your risk is to that of people who never smoked. And the more you smoked and the more recently you quit, the closer your risk is to that of current smokers.

As you examine the charts in the Extra Help section, you should notice a number of things. Looking across the rows lets you compare the chances of dying from different causes at a given age. This helps to put each cause of death in perspective—for example, you can see how the chance of dying from a heart attack compares to the chance of dying from lung cancer or to the chance of dying from all causes combined. Looking down the columns, you can see how risk changes with age. For most causes, the chance of dying increases steadily with age. So don't just focus on one number—look at the numbers around it, too.

Finally, by comparing the numbers for current smokers and people who never smoked, you can get a good sense of how much smoking increases your chance of dying. As you'll see, smoking makes a really big difference for some risks. For both men and women, at all ages, smoking greatly increases the chance of dying from heart attack, lung cancer, COPD, and all causes combined; it increases the chance of death from stroke and pneumonia too, but to a lesser extent.

In other cases, such as accidents or prostate cancer or AIDS, smoking does not make a difference. This makes sense: there is no biological reason that smoking would affect these causes. But if you look at the charts carefully, you'll see that smokers are a little *less* likely to die from some causes than people who never smoked. For example, the chance of a 75-year-old man dying from prostate cancer in the next 10 years is 19 in 1,000 for men who never smoked, but only 15 in 1,000 for men who currently smoke. Does that mean smoking protects you from prostate cancer? No, these small differences reflect the fact that these men die from only one cause—and since smoking increases their chance of dying from something like a heart attack or lung cancer (by a lot), that leaves fewer men to die from causes such as prostate cancer.

For smoking, the message is clear: it really increases your chance of dying. In fact, being a current smoker has the same effect on the risk of death from all causes combined as adding about 5 to 10 years of age. For example, the risk of death for a 55-year-old man who currently smokes is 178 out of 1,000, about the same as the risk for a 65-year-old who has never smoked (176 out of 1,000).

When you use the charts, be careful to choose the one for your sex. And then be careful to look at the right rows, choosing the one for your age and for whether you have never smoked or smoke now. If you use the wrong chart or look at the wrong rows, you'll get the wrong information.

Let's make sure you're using the charts correctly. For the following quiz, use the full risk charts in the Extra Help section (pages 128–129):

For Mr. Jones, the correct answer is c. Mr. Jones's chance of dying from lung cancer in the next 10 years is 89 in 1,000. If you answered 4 in 1,000, you looked at the wrong row of the chart (you found the number for men who have never smoked rather than the number for current smokers). If you said 55 in 1,000, you mistakenly used the chart for women who currently smoke.

For Mrs. Smith, the correct answer is a. Mrs. Smith's chance of dying from colon cancer in the next 10 years is 1 in 1,000. Note that her smoking history didn't matter—the chance of colon cancer death is not affected by smoking. If you answered 4 in 1,000, you probably looked at the wrong column of the chart (this is her chance of dying from breast cancer).

For Mr. Wilson, the correct answer is c. If Mr. Wilson still smoked, his chance of dying from a heart attack in the next 10 years would be 41 in 1,000. Because he quit, his chance will be lower. But because he smoked for a long time and quit only recently, the chance will still be pretty close to that of a current smoker, so we think the best guess is 31 in 1,000. Answer b (24 in 1,000) is also in the range between the nonsmoker and current smoker risks. But with Mr. Wilson's long history of smoking and his relatively short smoke-free time, it is unlikely that his risk dropped to this level. If you chose the answer 19 in 1,000, you looked at the row for people who never smoked.

Before you proceed to part two, be sure that you're comfortable reading the risk charts. These charts put the risk of death in perspective in a number of ways: comparing the chance of death across diseases, at different points in the life span, and in the context of all causes combined. They also send a strong message about how risk is increased by smoking.

Questions to Ask When Interpreting Risk

Throughout these first three chapters, we've emphasized the key questions you should ask when you're trying to make sense of messages about health risks. Here's a brief summary:

Risk of what?   Understand what the outcome is (getting a disease, dying from a disease, developing a symptom), and consider how bad it is.

How big is the risk?   Find out your chance of experiencing the outcome. If you hear about the number of people who experience an outcome, always ask, "Out of how many?" You need to know how many people could have experienced the outcome in order to calculate your own chance. Also ask, "What is the time frame?" Is the time frame for the risk the next year, the next 10 years, or a lifetime?

Because there are many ways to express the same risk, it's useful to put information in a consistent format. Our choice would be "___ out of 1,000 people over 10 years."

To get the full picture, we also suggest that you reframe the risk: for example, if 5 out of 1,000 people will die over 10 years, it is also true that 995 out of 1,000 will not die.

Does the risk information reasonably apply to me?   Determine whether the message is based on studies of people like you (people of your age and sex, people whose health is like yours).

How does this risk compare with other risks?   Get some perspective by asking about other risks you face so that you can develop a sense of just how big (or small) this particular risk really is.

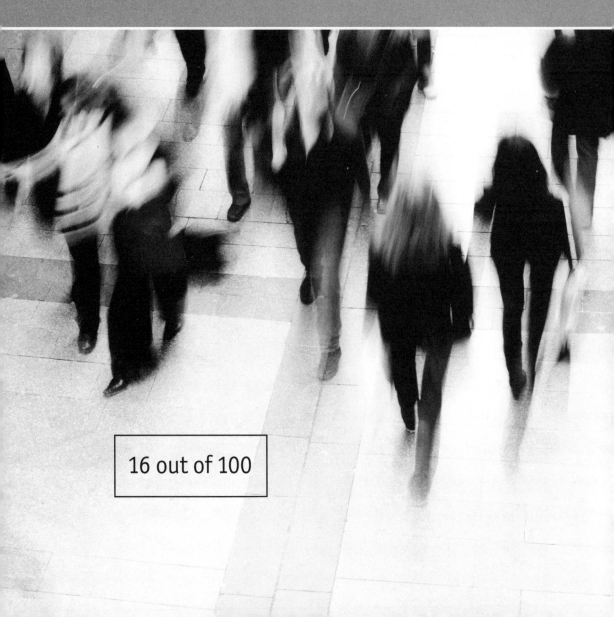

can i reduce my risk?

16 out of 100

judging the benefit of a health intervention

So far, you've been learning about the risk of getting or dying from a disease. But most messages are about how you can reduce those risks; that is, most messages focus on benefit. The word *benefit* refers to how much a risk is reduced by taking an action. Whatever the action is—taking medicine, having surgery, or changing your lifestyle—the formula is the same. You start out with a specific chance of something happening (the outcome), you take the action, and then, you hope, you have a lower chance of experiencing that outcome.

The lessons you learned about risk in part one of this book also apply to messages about risk reduction (that is, benefit), although these messages add some new challenges. As an example of a risk reduction message, we'll use a drug ad, simply because these ads have become so common. But what you learn will apply to any message about reducing risk.

In this section, we'll review risk reduction using an advertisement for Zocor, a drug used to lower a person's cholesterol level in order to reduce the chance of dying from a heart attack.

Before we go further, we'd like to make a few things clear. First, we chose this ad not because it is particularly egregious (in fact, it is probably better than the typical drug ad) but because it illustrates some common advertising tactics. Second, we did *not* choose this ad because we work for a drug company. We have no ties to any pharmaceutical company, and we use the trade name Zocor only to be consistent with the ad itself. Most important, we are not suggesting that you either use or avoid this drug. We just want to prepare you to make your own decisions.

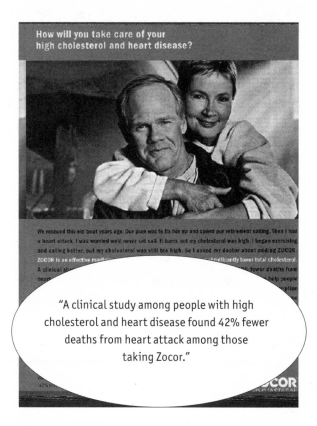

According to the ad, the man in the picture had a heart attack and has now found out that he has high cholesterol. He is worried about the future and wants to reduce his risk of another heart attack. The ad says that the medicine Zocor can help him. The white oval highlights the main message about how Zocor will change his risk. What does it mean?

As you know from the preceding chapters, the first two questions you should ask when you see a message about a risk are these:

Risk of what?   (What is the outcome?)
How big is the risk?   (What is the chance that you will experience the outcome, and over what time frame?)

You should ask similar questions when you see messages about risk reduction. The modified questions about risk reduction are the following:

Reduced risk of what?

How big is the risk reduction?

Look at the ad to try to answer these questions about Zocor:

Does the ad say that Zocor changes the chance of having a heart attack or the chance of dying from one? **QUIZ**
a. Having a heart attack
b. Dying from a heart attack
How much does Zocor change the risk?
a. From 1,000 in 1,000 to 580 in 1,000
b. From 100 in 1,000 to 58 in 1,000
c. From 10 in 1,000 to 5.8 in 1,000
d. Can't tell

The correct answer to the first question is b. The ad is clear on this point: it concerns a change in the risk of dying from a heart attack. It doesn't discuss how bad this risk is, but that's okay—it's obvious that dying from a heart attack is very bad. The ad, however, is not clear about the time frame. It turns out that the risk reduction reported (the benefit of taking Zocor) was calculated over a period of about 5 years.

The correct answer to the second question is d. Unfortunately, the main part of the ad doesn't tell you the chance of a fatal heart attack if you don't take Zocor compared to the chance if you do take Zocor (although the fine print contains some of this information). This is an important omission, and we'll come back to it in a little while.

You should ask one other question as you read the ad. You encountered it in earlier chapters, but once again we're modifying it to focus on risk reduction:

Does the risk reduction information reasonably apply to me?   The ad does a relatively good job here. The message is about people with both high cholesterol and heart disease. If you have heart disease but normal cholesterol, or high cholesterol but no heart disease, this ad does not apply to you. What about age and sex? On these points, the ad is not clear. You have to go to the original article published in the medical journal to learn about who was actually in the study.[1] It turns out that the people who participated in the study were mostly men in their early 60s. Overall, however, the ages of the participants ranged from 35 to 70, so the information probably applies to people as young as 35 and as old as 70. Only 20 percent of the people in the study were women. So women should be less confident that the benefit information applies to them.

Overall, this ad, like many messages about how actions can reduce risk, is sketchy on important details. Because people's minds have a tendency to fill in missing details, you might assume that the risk the drug addresses is big (why else would the drug be advertised?) and that it applies to all readers. The questions we've just reviewed point out the missing facts and are outlined in the quick summary in the Extra Help section of this book (pages 117–119). Whenever you're faced with risk reduction messages, we encourage you to review the quick summary to help you see which facts are missing.

Now that we've established what risk is being reduced, let's focus on how big the risk reduction might be for those who use Zocor. Here's how the ad describes the benefit of Zocor: "A clinical study among people with high cholesterol and heart disease found 42 percent fewer deaths from heart attack among those taking Zocor."

When someone tells you something like this—"42 percent fewer deaths"—the most important question to ask is "42 percent fewer than what?" Unless you know what number is being lowered by 42 percent, it's impossible to judge how big the change is.

Thinking about risk reduction is like deciding when to use a coupon at a store. Imagine that you have a coupon for 50 percent off any one purchase. You go to the store to buy a pack of gum, which costs 50 cents, and a large Thanksgiving turkey, which costs $35.00. Will you use the coupon for the gum or for the turkey? Most people would use the coupon for the turkey. Here's why:

Item	Regular Price	"50% Off" Sale Price	Savings
Gum	$0.50	$0.25	$0.25
Turkey	$35.00	$17.50	$17.50

In both cases, you save 50 percent. But with a cheap item, you save very little (25 cents); with an expensive item, you save a lot ($17.50). Obviously, to know what a discount means, you must know the regular price. The same is true in health care: "50 percent fewer deaths" is a different number in reference to a rare cause of death than it is in reference to a common cause. To understand how big a difference an action could make, you must find out the *starting* and *modified risks*—called *absolute risks* in the jargon of researchers. With the store coupon, the starting and modified risks are the regular price and the sales price. In a study about a medical treatment, the starting and modified risks are the chances of an outcome in the untreated and treated groups (that is, those who did not take the drug versus those who did).

QUIZ

Imagine that you are a typical 70-year-old woman who has never smoked. Consider two drugs. Both drugs lower the chance of dying from a disease by 50 percent, and they are equally safe. One works on cervical cancer, and the other works on heart attacks. Which drug is more likely to help keep you alive?

HINT: Refer to the risk charts in the Extra Help section to learn the risk of death for each disease.

    a. Drug for cervical cancer
    b. Drug for heart attack

The correct answer is b. For a typical 70-year-old woman, the chance of dying from cervical cancer in the next 10 years is 1 in 1,000. Her chance of dying from a heart attack is much larger: 46 in 1,000 (remember, she has never smoked, so when you consult the risk chart, you should be looking in the row for women who have never smoked). So she is much more likely to benefit from the drug that lowers the chance of heart attack death.

Let's go back to the original Zocor ad and figure out what "42 percent fewer deaths from heart attack" really means. In (very) small print at the bottom of the ad, the following statement appears:

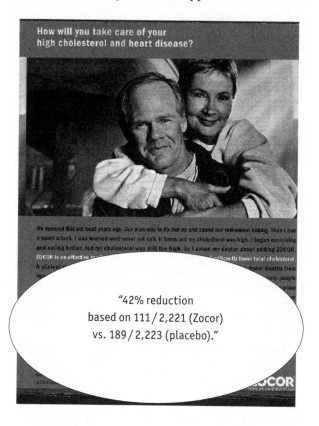

How will you take care of your high cholesterol and heart disease?

"42% reduction based on 111 / 2,221 (Zocor) vs. 189 / 2,223 (placebo)."

This statement provides the data you need to answer the question "42 percent fewer than what?" It tells you the information needed to calculate the starting risk: the number of people in the untreated (placebo) group who had the outcome divided by the total number of people in the untreated group (189 / 2,223). This is to the manufacturer's credit. It would have been nice if they had done the division for you, but at least the information is there. And, in fact, the ad also presents the information needed to calculate the modified risk: the number of people in the treated (Zocor) group who had the outcome divided by the total number of people in the treated group (111 / 2,221).

In any event, whenever you are given the data in this way (for example, 111 / 2,221 versus 189 / 2,223), we suggest that you do the division yourself. It involves two calculations, one for the group of people who were not treated with Zocor but instead took a placebo (a sugar pill that has no effect), and another for the group of people who took Zocor. Here's how we did the math:

Starting risk = risk of heart attack death for people in the placebo group

$$= \frac{189 \text{ heart attack deaths}}{2{,}223 \text{ people who took a placebo}} = 8.5\%$$

Modified risk = risk of heart attack death for people in the Zocor group

$$= \frac{111 \text{ heart attack deaths}}{2{,}221 \text{ people who took Zocor}} = 5.0\%$$

So taking Zocor lowered the chance of dying from a heart attack in the next 5 years from 8.5 percent (the starting risk) to 5.0 percent (the modified risk). The following graph may help you to understand this difference better.

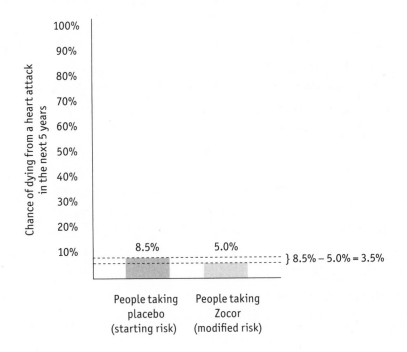

Guess what 8.5 percent reduced by 42 percent is? It turns out to be 5.0 percent. The benefit of Zocor, "42 percent fewer deaths," means that if you have heart disease and high cholesterol and you take Zocor, your chance of dying from a heart attack is 42 percent lower than it would be if you didn't take Zocor. Another way to think about how Zocor changes your risk is to imagine a "42 percent off" sale in which the regular price is 8.5 percent, the sale price is 5.0 percent, and your savings equal 3.5 percent. (The Learn More box on page 45 shows how to do the calculations for each way of talking about risk reduction and provides the standard statistical language.)

These ways of describing a benefit can get confusing, for doctors and patients alike. We think that the best way to understand risk reduction information is to determine what your risk is if you do not take the medicine (or other treatment) and then compare it with your risk if you do—specifically, you need to look at your starting and modified risks, side by side. Here's the message rewritten in this way:

> "For men with heart disease and high cholesterol, Zocor reduces the 5-year chance of dying of a heart attack from 8.5 percent to 5.0 percent."

Does this sound less impressive than the original "42 percent fewer deaths" version? Most people say yes. This is another example of framing (explained in chapter 1). The same information—the extent to which Zocor lowers the risk of dying from a heart attack—sounds very different depending on how it is expressed ("42 percent lower" or "8.5 percent versus 5.0 percent").[2]

To be sure you understand these different expressions, try this quiz:

QUIZ Drug X is for people with high blood pressure. In a study, it reduced the chance of having a stroke over the next 10 years from 8% to 4%. Which of these statements is true?

    a. The starting risk = 8%

    b. The modified risk = 4%

    c. The drug lowers risk by 50%

    d. The drug lowers risk by 4 percentage points

    e. All of the above

Learn More

Calculating Risk Reductions

So which is it? Does Zocor lower risk by 42 percent or 3.5 percent? Actually, both figures are correct. They are just two different ways of framing the answer. The 42 percent statistic is a *relative risk reduction*—in other words, it tells you how much lower a 5.0 percent risk is, relative to an 8.5 percent risk. Calculating the relative risk reduction involves division:

Relative risk reduction

$$= \frac{\text{starting risk} - \text{modified risk}}{\text{starting risk}}$$

$$= \frac{\text{risk of heart attack (placebo group)} - \text{risk of heart attack (Zocor group)}}{\text{risk of heart attack (placebo group)}}$$

$$= \frac{8.5\% - 5.0\%}{8.5\%} = 0.42 = 42\%$$

The 3.5 percent statistic is an *absolute risk reduction*—in other words, it tells you how much lower a 5 percent risk is than an 8.5 percent risk in absolute terms. Calculating the absolute risk reduction involves subtraction:

Absolute risk reduction

$$= \text{starting risk} - \text{modified risk}$$
$$= \text{risk of heart attack (placebo group)} - \text{risk of heart attack (Zocor group)}$$
$$= 8.5\% - 5.0\% = 3.5\%$$

Some people prefer to express this statistic as a "3.5 percentage point difference" to make it clear that they are describing an absolute risk reduction. (The expression "3.5 percent reduction" could be taken to mean either a relative or an absolute risk reduction.)

The correct answer is e. All of the statements are true.

Now that you have good information about the starting and modified risks, you are faced with deciding whether this difference is big or small (or big enough to make it worth taking a pill). This is not an easy question, and the decision can be tricky. While it's tempting to say that the difference between an 8.5 percent chance and a 5.0 percent chance of heart attack death over the next 5 years is pretty small, we'd say that it is actually pretty big. Why? Because, as you can see in the risk charts, heart attacks are a major cause of death for men and women, smokers and nonsmokers alike. And only a few drugs have been shown to reduce heart attack death at all.

So be careful about dismissing the importance of anything that can reduce a major cause of death (we'll have more to say about that in the next chapter). Most people don't have a good sense of how well drugs typically work. This is not surprising, since people rarely get to see the relevant information. We hope that this will change. Specifically, we hope that the U.S. Food and Drug Administration and others will help make drug benefit information more readily available to consumers (and that consumers will start demanding this information!) so that over time people will learn to better appreciate what constitutes a sizable benefit. In general, any treatment that reduces deaths from a major cause such as heart attack, even by a small amount (like 1 percentage point), is probably worth considering.

It's no coincidence that drug ads—when they do provide some data about how well drugs work (which is not very often)—typically present risk reduction information in a format such as "42 percent fewer" or "42 percent lower." Why? Because expressing benefit as a relative change makes even small risk reductions sound big. And it may contribute to an unrealistic sense about how effective various medications are. We think that failing to ask, "Fewer than what?" or "Lower than what?" is the single most important omission in trying to understand messages about risk reduction. If you hear only an expression of relative change, but not the starting and modified risks, you don't have the data you really need to appreciate the magnitude of the benefit. When you've heard only a large number (like "42 percent lower"), you may tend to overestimate the size of the benefit.

A great way to highlight the information you need to understand how well a drug or other intervention works is to create a table like this one:

Outcome (Time frame: over ___ years)	Starting Risk (Untreated group)	Modified Risk (Treated group)

Our advice is to try filling in the table so that you can compare the starting and modified risks side by side. If you're being advised to consider a major intervention, you should ask those offering the advice to complete the table for you. If they can't—and if you can't find a way to complete it yourself—you need to be very cautious about the intervention. If you're unable to fill in the table, it means that you don't know what the intervention really offers. Sometimes you do have to make important decisions in the face of great uncertainty. But that is very different from making decisions under the illusion that you know something when you don't.

For practice, try reading the following "news story" about some hypothetical research findings concerning a (fictional) new drug:

Promising New Drug Hailed

Washington, D.C.—Researchers announced the results of a long-awaited study of Argentex, a drug designed to prevent prostate cancer. In the study, 1,000 men ages 45 to 75 were randomly assigned to take either Argentex or a sugar pill called a placebo. The men were followed for 4 years. Men taking Argentex had a 40 percent lower risk of developing prostate cancer. Lead scientist Bernard Womba described the findings as "extremely promising" and predicted that the drug would be in wide use shortly.

What were the starting and modified risks in the study showing that Argentex reduced risk by 40%?

	Starting Risk (Placebo group)	Modified Risk (Argentex group)
a.	0.05%	0.03%
b.	5%	3%
c.	50%	30%
d.	0.010%	0.006%
e.	1%	0.6%
f.	10%	6%

Sorry—this is another trick question. The answer is that you just can't tell. All the answers listed in the quiz are possible, as are many other answers. But you can't select the "right one" because key information—the actual starting risk—is missing. You may not have enjoyed this quiz: it's annoying to be asked to do the impossible. But what's really annoying is how often this scenario occurs in real life. As you begin to look for starting and modified risk numbers, you may discover that they can be very hard to find. Even articles in medical journals sometimes omit these basic statistics and provide only information about relative change, using expressions like "40 percent lower."

For a little more practice, here's a table for another fictional drug, this one called Pridclo. This drug is for people who already have heart disease (that is, they have already had a heart attack). After you read the table, try taking the quiz that follows.

Outcome (Time frame: over 2 years)	Starting Risk (Placebo group)	Modified Risk (Pridclo group)
Dying from a heart attack or stroke	3%	2%

For people with heart disease, who is less likely to die from a heart attack or stroke in the next 2 years: someone who takes Pridclo or someone who takes a placebo?

  a. Someone who takes Pridclo
  b. Someone who takes a placebo
  c. Can't tell

Pridclo reduces the risk of dying from a heart attack or stroke by about 33 percent.

  a. True
  b. False
  c. Can't tell

What is the difference between the starting risk and the modified risk with Pridclo?

  a. 3 percentage points
  b. 2 percentage points
  c. 1 percentage point

The correct answer to the first question is a. If you've read the table correctly, you'll see that people with heart disease can reduce their chance of dying from a heart attack or stroke in the next 2 years from 3 percent to 2 percent by taking Pridclo. In other words, for every 100 people with heart disease who take Pridclo, there will be 1 less death in the next 2 years.

The correct answer to the second question is a. The statement is true. But since you know the starting and modified risks, you can appreciate that the 33 percent risk reduction corresponds to a change from 3 in 100 to 2 in 100:

$$\frac{\text{starting risk} - \text{modified risk}}{\text{starting risk}} = \frac{3-2}{3} = \frac{1}{3} = 0.33 = 33\%$$

The correct answer to the third question is c. Pridclo lowers risk of heart attack or stroke by 1 percentage point. Both the statements "33 percent lower" and "1 percentage point lower" correctly summarize the benefit of taking Pridclo. We think that the least ambiguous and most transparent way to describe the benefit is to show the starting and modified risks side by side, as we did in the table. Once you have those two statistics, you have the full picture (and in fact you can calculate the absolute risk reduction or the relative risk reduction, as shown in the Learn More box on page 45).

Why Starting Risk Matters

Starting risk determines how big the benefit of an action can be. People who start at a high risk usually stand to gain much more from taking action than people who start at a low risk.

Let's take a closer look at the Zocor ad on page 38. This ad describes the benefit of taking the medicine for people with heart disease and high cholesterol. Do you think that the benefit might be different for people without heart disease?

QUIZ Who has a greater chance of dying from a heart attack in the next 5 years?

a. Men like Mr. Smith, a 55-year-old with very high cholesterol who has had two heart attacks already

b. Men like Mr. Jones, a 55-year-old with mildly elevated cholesterol and no heart disease

The answer, of course, is a. So who is more likely to benefit from taking Zocor? The answer is **a** again. Men like Smith start out at higher risk than men like Jones. If Zocor lowers the risk of heart attack death by 42 percent for both groups, the benefit is greater for high-risk people. (Remember the earlier example: a coupon for 50 percent off the price is more valuable when you're purchasing an expensive item like a turkey than it is when you're buying something cheap like gum.) Let's use a table to look at the numbers.

Outcome (Time frame: over 5 years)	Starting Risk (Placebo group)	Modified Risk (Zocor group)	Starting Risk Minus Modified Risk (Change with Zocor)
Men with heart disease (like Smith) dying from a heart attack	8.5%	5.0%	3.5 percentage points lower
Men without heart disease (like Jones) dying from a heart attack	2.0%	1.2%	0.8 percentage point lower

Where you start matters! The higher your starting risk, the more you stand to benefit from treatments that reduce that risk. And the lower your starting risk, the less you stand to benefit even from the best intervention. This is true for heart disease and any other disease.

To understand why, think about the nature of an illness or health condition. In general, the sicker you are from a disease, the more likely you are to have a bad outcome related to that disease, such as a complication, hospitalization, or even death. Consequently, sicker people have a lot to gain from reducing their risk of a bad outcome: their starting risk is really high, so there's much more risk to reduce.

Now consider people who are only mildly sick. They may still have a bad outcome, but it's much less likely than it would be for very sick people. Since the starting risk of mildly sick people is low to begin with, even an effective intervention can help only a little, at best. There just isn't that much risk to reduce.

As an example, the following table summarizes the chance that different groups of people will experience a bad outcome without treatment (look at the starting risk numbers) or with treatment (look at the modified risk numbers). For this example, we assert that the treatment lowers risk by 50 percent. This 50 percent reduction translates into benefits of varying size, depending on each group's starting risk, as shown in the last column of the table.

How Sick?	Starting Risk	Modified Risk	Relative Change (% lower risk)	Starting Risk Minus Modified Risk
Very sick	50%	25%	50%	25 percentage points lower
Moderately sick	10%	5%	50%	5 percentage points lower
Mildly sick	5%	2.5%	50%	2.5 percentage points lower
Not sick	1%	0.5%	50%	0.5 percentage point lower

The table illustrates a key point. The size of the benefit you might experience from a treatment depends on your starting risk. The same 50 percent reduction in risk translates to a much bigger benefit for people who are very sick compared to that for people who are well. As a general rule, sicker patients stand to gain more from treatments than do people who are less sick.

Thus, when a study indicates that a treatment has a good chance of working, you must be cautious about assuming that these results will apply to you. You need to be sure that the study involved people who are similar to you—not just in terms of age and sex but also in terms of their starting risk. Remember that if you aren't at all like the people in the study, you can't assume that you would experience the same benefit as the study participants. But the more you are like the people in the study, the more likely it is that you face the same starting risk and would experience the same benefit.

Starting Risks Can Be Hard to Find

Even though they are crucial to know, starting risks are often missing. We—and others—have documented this problem in several systematic studies of medical journals, medical journal press releases, news stories, and ads. Here's what has been found:

Nearly 70 percent of articles published in major medical journals did not include starting risks in the abstract (the most widely read part of the article), and one-third did not include starting risks anywhere in the article.[3]

Forty-five percent of the press releases issued by major medical journals did not include starting risks, which may be one reason these statistics are often missing in news stories.[4]

News reports of medical research often do not contain starting risks.[5]

Direct-to-consumer prescription drug ads rarely provide starting risks— only 3 percent of the ads we studied contained them.[6]

If you start to pay close attention to drug ads and news stories, you'll be amazed at how often you are told that a risk is "40 percent lower" without ever being told "lower than what?" (the starting risk).

Questions to Ask about Risk Reduction

As this chapter explained, there are three key questions you should ask when you hear a message about how some action can reduce your risk:

Reduced risk of what?   Understand what outcome is being changed (getting a disease, dying from a disease, developing a symptom), and decide how much you care about it.

How big is the risk reduction?   Find out your chance of experiencing the outcome if you don't take an action (such as taking a medication or changing your lifestyle) and your chance if you do take the action. In other words, know your starting and modified risks. This is especially important if you hear a message like "drug X lowers your risk by 42 percent." Always ask, "Lower than what?" Unless you know your starting risk (the "lower than what" part), the message really tells you nothing.

Does the risk information reasonably apply to me?   Learn whether the message is based on studies of people like you (people of your age and sex, people whose health is like yours). The more you are like the participants in the studies, the more likely you are to face the same starting risk and experience the same benefit.

not all benefits are equal: **5** understand the outcome

The Zocor ad introduced in chapter 4 mentions two benefits for people who have high cholesterol and heart disease: the drug lowers cholesterol levels, and it reduces the chance of death from a heart attack. The drug has other benefits as well: it reduces the chance of a nonfatal heart attack, and it lowers the chance of developing a weakened heart—a condition known as heart failure—which makes sense, since fewer heart attacks mean less weakening.

All the things Zocor affects—cholesterol levels, the chance of fatal and nonfatal heart attacks, and heart failure—are called outcomes. As you've learned, the benefit of drugs or other interventions is measured in terms of how they affect outcomes. In chapter 4, we listed some questions that you should ask whenever you hear a message about how an action can reduce your risk. The first question to ask is this: "Reduced risk of what?" The answer is the outcome.

Only when you understand the outcome under consideration does it make sense to ask the second question: "How big is the risk reduction?" Without a clear picture of the seriousness or importance of the outcome, you can't decide if the risk reduction is big enough to make the action worthwhile. In fact, if you don't care about the outcome, there's no reason to even bother learning the size of the benefit.

So how do you decide if you care about the outcome? The following illustration organizes outcomes according to their direct impact on you. We call it the *pyramid of benefit*. At the bottom are things that don't have a direct impact on you—for example, laboratory measurements, blood tests, and X-rays. You don't directly experience or feel these outcomes; for instance, you don't feel any different if your cholesterol level is really low or really high. On the pyramid, these kinds of outcomes are called *surrogate outcomes.*

As you move up the pyramid, you encounter *patient outcomes,* where the impact of the outcomes becomes increasingly direct: you clearly feel symptoms such as pain and nausea, for example, and you directly experience events such as being hospitalized, requiring nursing home care, or needing an operation. And since it is hard to think of anything that has a more direct impact on you, death appears at the top of the pyramid. Because the pyramid may be useful in helping you decide which outcomes you care about, the following sections examine it in some detail.

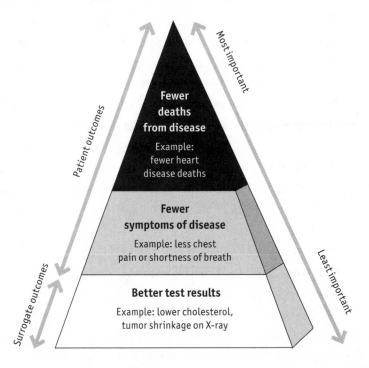

Better Test Results

Many medical interventions change surrogate outcomes, such as laboratory measurements of cholesterol levels or X-ray results that measure bone density. Since you cannot directly feel these surrogate outcomes, why should you care about them? The reason is that these outcomes often "stand in" for, or represent, patient outcomes higher on the pyramid. A surrogate is something that stands in for something else.

Unfortunately, surrogate outcomes often do a poor job of "standing in" for patient outcomes. Keep this in mind! Even if a drug improves a surrogate outcome, it doesn't mean that the drug will improve a corresponding patient outcome. Judging benefit based solely on a surrogate outcome requires a big leap of faith.

As an example, consider a drug that has been demonstrated to lower cholesterol levels (a surrogate outcome). A host of medical studies have shown that lower cholesterol levels are linked to fewer heart attacks (a patient outcome). Does this mean that the drug will reduce the number of heart attacks? It may—but it may not. Improving a surrogate outcome does not automatically mean improving a patient outcome. (See the Learn More box on page 58.)

Consider a health message, adapted from a real ad for an osteoporosis drug, claiming that "drug X improves bone density by 35 percent." (Osteoporosis means thinning bones.) This improvement may sound pretty encouraging. But let's take a closer look. To start, ask yourself, "What is the outcome?" The answer is greater bone mineral density. Unless you know what bone density means, the 35 percent statistic won't matter to you. Bone density is a way of gauging how strong bones are. But you don't feel bone density—it's a surrogate outcome. The only reason we care about bone density is because weak, thin bones are more apt to fracture. And bone fractures—something people directly experience—are important: they hurt, and they can leave people disabled. For the elderly, hip fractures in particular are often the first step toward institutionalization or even death.

But what if drug X improved your bone density (measured by a T-score) but did not lower your chance of a hip fracture, the most disabling kind of bone fracture? This is not so far-fetched. Lots of things other than bone

Learn More

When Surrogate Outcomes Mislead

There are many examples of beneficial changes in surrogate outcomes that fail to translate into beneficial changes in patient outcomes. Let's look at the famous example of clofibrate, a cholesterol-lowering drug that actually *increased* heart attack risk. Clofibrate did a good job of lowering cholesterol levels. However, many physicians were shocked in the 1970s when a large randomized trial (a "gold standard" study) showed that people with initially high cholesterol who took clofibrate ended up with lower cholesterol levels but were *more likely* to have a fatal heart attack than people who were given a placebo.

Hormone replacement therapy (HRT) for women after menopause provides a more recent example. HRT involves taking estrogen. Because estrogen raises the level of "good" cholesterol (HDL), and high HDL levels are linked to lower heart attack risk, many physicians made a leap of faith and assumed for years that HRT would lead to fewer heart attacks. But when a large randomized trial—the Women's Health Initiative—was finally conducted, it found that women who took estrogen ended up with higher HDL levels but nevertheless had slightly more heart attacks than women who were given a placebo.[1] In other words, despite the surrogate outcome getting better, the patient outcome got worse.

There are three general reasons why beneficial changes in surrogate outcomes fail to translate into beneficial changes in patient outcomes:

(1) The link between the surrogate outcome and the patient outcome is weak. For example, let's say you hear of a new cancer drug that shrinks tumors. You cannot assume that tumor shrinkage will translate into living longer or even feeling better. Tumor shrinkage may be followed by a period of rapid tumor growth, or the shrinkage may happen in an unimportant area that doesn't affect your health. Or the size of the tumor may not be nearly as important as whether or not the tumor has spread to other parts of the body.

(2) The treatment that improves the surrogate outcome may affect the body in many ways. For example, hormone replacement—in addition to raising good cholesterol—makes the blood more likely to clot. More clotting leads to more heart attacks. Only by measuring the patient outcome (heart attacks) were we able to

learn the net result of hormone replacement therapy: HRT increased the chance that a woman would have a heart attack.

(3) The surrogate outcome may not be the actual cause of the patient outcome. Although studies may show a link between a surrogate outcome and a patient outcome, this link might be the result of some other factor (scientists call this a *confounding factor*). Consequently, even if the treatment changes the surrogate outcome a lot, it may not change the patient outcome at all. For example, many studies that observed people who took antioxidant vitamins such as vitamin C or E found that these people had fewer heart attacks. But a large randomized trial showed that these vitamins didn't work to reduce heart attacks (even though antioxidant vitamin levels in the blood of participants increased). This study proved that there was something else about the people who took vitamins (such as eating a healthier diet or not smoking) that explained why they had fewer heart attacks. Taking vitamins improved the surrogate outcome (it increased vitamin levels in the blood), but higher antioxidant levels apparently did not lead to fewer heart attacks.

density affect your chance of fracturing a bone, including factors that increase your chance of falling, such as poor vision, poor balance, or even how your house is set up (lots of clutter, throw rugs). And increased bone density is not the only ingredient of bone strength—for example, bone architecture (the underlying structure of the bone) may matter even more. As it turns out, although many drugs improve bone density, few have been shown to reduce hip fractures.

If drug X works only on the surrogate outcome (bone density), but this benefit does not translate into the corresponding patient outcome (fewer hip fractures), you would be wise to be hesitant about exposing yourself to the cost, inconvenience, and potential side effects of the drug. This would be true no matter how big an effect drug X has on the surrogate outcome.

You cannot reliably assume that improving a surrogate outcome will translate into better health. Nevertheless, you will hear about surrogate outcomes all the time (especially in drug ads), because they are easier and faster to measure than patient outcomes: a drug may lower cholesterol levels right away, but it will take years to see whether the drug really results in fewer heart attacks. If you hear about a medical intervention that improves a surrogate outcome, ask this question: "Has the intervention also been shown to have a beneficial effect on what people experience or feel?"

QUIZ A study in a major medical journal reports that a new drug can shrink liver tumors. What is the most important additional information you would want to know?

a. How much the tumors shrink
b. Whether people feel better or live longer

The correct answer is b. Tumor shrinkage is a surrogate outcome. It may translate into longer, better lives—but it may not. Unfortunately, we have many examples of cancer drugs that shrink tumors but do not extend life (some even shorten it). Surrogate outcomes matter only to the extent that they improve the corresponding patient outcome (the outcome they stand in for). So knowing how much the drug shrinks the tumors isn't really important—unless the drug makes people feel better or live longer.

Now you know why we consider surrogate outcomes to be less important than patient outcomes.

Fewer Symptoms of Disease

The next step on the pyramid addresses the benefit of fewer symptoms of disease. Symptoms are the disease-related sensations people feel. The most familiar symptom is pain: headache, back pain, joint pain, chest pain. Many other common symptoms can be very unpleasant though not painful: upset stomach, shortness of breath, lightheadedness, and runny nose, for instance.

Most people do not need to think long and hard about the importance of interventions that make them feel better when they are sick. That's why we believe that a reduction of symptoms is a very important outcome. For most people, symptom relief matters so much that they are eager to get to the next questions and ask for the numbers: "How big is the benefit? That is, how likely is it that I will feel better if I take this action? And how much better will I feel?"

In fact, some people wouldn't even bother asking about the numbers. People with symptoms can often see for themselves whether the intervention works, by trying it. For example, if your headache doesn't improve after taking a headache medicine, you may decide that the pills don't work. Alternatively, if the headache goes away completely in twenty minutes, you'll probably decide that the drug is a winner.

Mr. Smith started taking a drug for restless legs. After 12 weeks, he says that his legs feel much better. Can you be sure that the improvement is a result of the drug?

QUIZ

    a. Yes

    b. No

The correct answer is b. Symptom improvement is not a foolproof test of benefit. Some people feel better just because they do something. You may have heard of the *placebo effect:* people sometimes experience a benefit even when they take an ineffective sugar pill or when they receive a faked surgery. And some symptoms, by their very nature, wax and wane spontaneously. People with back pain know this quite well: on some days, their back feels great; on other days, it feels awful. These two factors—the placebo effect and spontaneous improvement—can lead people to judge an intervention as being beneficial when in fact it is not. For these reasons, the most trustworthy test of an intervention for current symptoms is a randomized trial—a true experiment, in which people are randomly given either the treatment or a placebo and then undergo a standardized symptom assessment. If the treatment works, the people who were randomly chosen to receive it will, on average, do better than those randomly chosen to receive the placebo.

Deciding whether a treatment works by trying it is possible, of course, only when you have symptoms—this strategy doesn't work with interven-

Learn More

When Symptom Improvement Isn't Enough

Requip—the first drug to treat restless legs syndrome—is a great example of how hard it can be to judge whether a drug is the reason you feel better. In the largest study of the drug, about 200 people with moderate to severe restless legs syndrome were given Requip.[2] After 12 weeks, about 70 percent (70 out of 100) of these people had substantial improvement. (This is the modified risk.) Does this mean that Requip works? No. Unless you can compare this improvement to what would have happened without Requip, you can't understand whether there is a benefit. That's why you need a comparison group.

The comparison group in this study consisted of 200 people with moderate to severe restless legs syndrome who were given a placebo. Interestingly, 55 percent (55 out of 100) of the placebo group also had substantial improvement. (This is the starting risk.) Based on this comparison, the benefit of taking Requip is the difference between 55 percent improvement and 70 percent improvement. In other words, given that so many people got better without any treatment, we can conclude that only 15 percent (15 out of 100) actually felt better because of the drug. When there is such a big placebo effect, it is really hard to know whether feeling better is in fact a result of the drug. Unfortunately, this can lead many people to continue to take a medication that isn't really helping them.

tions that are designed to reduce your risk of some future event. If you take Zocor, for example, you won't feel your "reduced risk" of a future fatal heart attack. The only way to gauge the benefit of interventions that reduce a future risk is to know the numbers: your starting and modified risks, as outlined in chapter 4.

Fewer Deaths from Disease

Because reducing the number of deaths from disease is a very important outcome, it appears at the top of the pyramid. There isn't a lot of ambiguity here—death is really important to most people. So interventions that reduce the number of deaths almost always matter (a lot) to people. But you

Learn More

Fewer Diagnoses of Disease: How Important?

The pyramid of benefit shows three categories of benefits that can result from medical interventions: fewer deaths, fewer symptoms, and better test results. But there is another category of benefit to consider: fewer diagnoses of disease. Some interventions reduce the chance that you will be diagnosed with a disease.

On the face of it, reducing your chance of being diagnosed with a disease sounds like a very desirable benefit—and it can be. But recognizing how important this benefit is can be surprisingly tricky. To understand why, try to decide where it fits on the pyramid of benefit.

Do fewer diagnoses of disease always mean fewer deaths? Certainly not. For most cancers and other serious diseases, diagnosis does not equal death.

Nor do fewer diagnoses always mean fewer symptoms of disease. That's because many diseases, especially in their milder forms, have no symptoms to begin with. For example, except in the most extreme cases, high blood pressure has no symptoms. Nor does mild type 2 diabetes, anemia, or kidney disease. These diagnoses are made by doing blood tests.

So sometimes fewer diagnoses simply mean better test results. But in those cases, the outcomes may not be very important. That's because test results are surrogate outcomes—and as we've discussed, surrogate outcomes are not always closely linked to patient outcomes. Not everyone with mildly abnormal test results develops severe abnormalities or symptoms. So preventing diseases that are diagnosed only by tests will not translate into a tangible benefit for everyone. The link between better test results and fewer symptoms is tenuous—and there may be no link between better test results and fewer deaths.

The point is that fewer diagnoses of disease can have a range of meanings. Some interventions that result in fewer diagnoses matter more than others. We think that, in general, the benefit of fewer diagnoses of diseases with symptoms is more important than the benefit of fewer diagnoses of diseases defined just by test results. To help yourself decide how much this benefit matters, ask: "Do fewer diagnoses mean that I will live longer? Or feel better? Or feel better longer? Or just have a better-looking medical record?"

should still go ahead and find out the numbers. You might be surprised: you might not care so much about an intervention that reduces a very rare cause of death, or even one that reduces a common cause of death by a very, very small amount.

We should also acknowledge that, in some cases, reducing the risk of death is not always the most desirable effect. For someone with terminal cancer or end-stage Alzheimer's, minimizing suffering—symptoms—may be more important than prolonging life.

In this chapter, we showed you how the pyramid of benefit can help you decide how much to care. Of course, the less you care about the outcome, the less important it is to bother thinking about the size of the benefit.

Pay attention to the outcome that is addressed in any health message—it may not be the one you care about most. When you hear about how a drug affects a blood test result, such as cholesterol or bone density scores, remember to keep your eyes on the prize: cholesterol, other lab tests, X-rays, and so on may matter. But they may not. Do people who take the drug live longer? Do they feel better? Or does the drug just make their test results look better? What really matters to you is how these things translate into how you feel, how they affect your chance of living the way you want to live, and whether they affect your chance of dying.

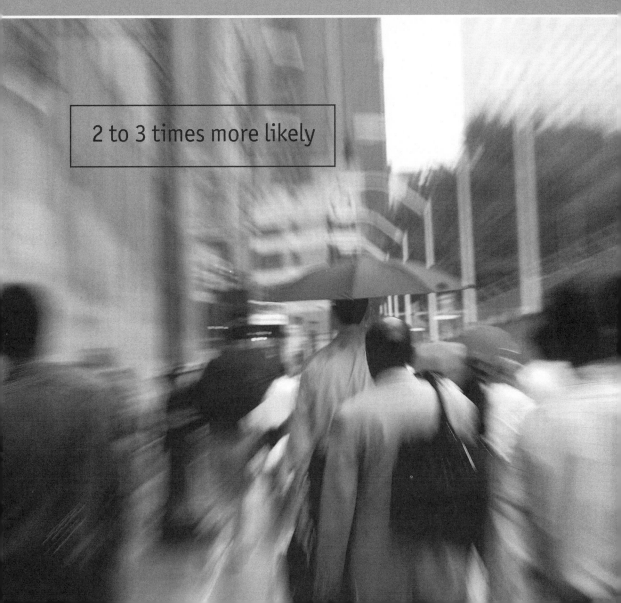

PART THREE

does risk reduction
have downsides?

2 to 3 times more likely

We have saved fivepence.
But at what cost?

Samuel Beckett, *All That Fall*

consider the downsides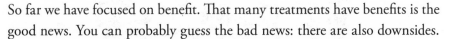

So far we have focused on benefit. That many treatments have benefits is the good news. You can probably guess the bad news: there are also downsides.

These downsides include side effects, cost, and inconvenience. We're not going to say much about cost and inconvenience. Cost, of course, varies widely—it depends on the type of treatment, whether you have insurance, and what kind of policy you have. You have to learn what the cost is to you and decide how much it matters.

Inconvenience includes a whole range of potential nuisances. Medical care can be time-consuming and annoying—you need to make phone calls (and wait while you're on hold), make appointments, go back for blood tests, fill out forms, get prescription refills, and so on. Again, you have to determine what the inconveniences will be and decide how much they matter.

In this chapter, we focus on side effects, the most important downsides you might experience.

All drugs and medical interventions have side effects. Although the benefit can be substantial, the side effects can be substantial too. And they may be so substantial that they overwhelm the benefit. We find it useful to think about two categories: *symptom side effects* and *life-threatening side effects*.

You should think about side effects the same way you've learned to think about benefit: be clear about the nature of the possible side effects of the intervention; and then, if any of them matter to you, get the numbers. This chapter lets you practice by using a few real drugs as examples. (We remind you again that we have no ties to any pharmaceutical company. Most important, we are not suggesting that you either use or avoid any of the drugs discussed.)

Let's begin with symptom side effects, those effects that are unpleasant or even painful but not life-threatening. Many, if not most, Americans have seen the luna moth that is the symbol of the sleeping pill Lunesta. Sepracor, the drug's manufacturer, spent over $250 million advertising the drug in 1 year. Here's one of the magazine ads:

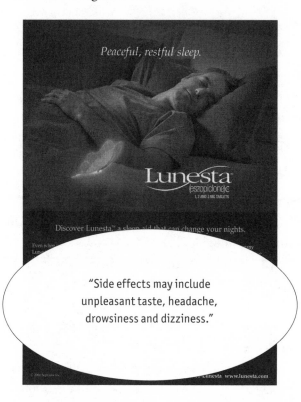

The U.S. Food and Drug Administration (FDA) requires that direct-to-consumer drug advertisements include a description of frequently occurring side effects. We've highlighted how this was done in the Lunesta ad. As you can see, four side effects are noted: unpleasant taste, headache, drowsiness, and dizziness.

If you care about any of these side effects, your next step is to get the numbers—to find out how often people taking the drug experience the side effects. Unfortunately, getting the numbers is not an easy task. This ad doesn't provide any of the statistics (in fact, they are not available even in the "patient information" that appears in small print on the page following the ad). All you get is a list of possible side effects. Without the numbers, how can you possibly decide whether to take the drug?

Consider one of the side effects listed for Lunesta, drowsiness. Here, drowsiness means feeling sleepy the next day (when you want to be awake and alert). Would you be happy if the pill helped you sleep better at night but made you feel drowsy the next day? What chance of next-day drowsiness would be acceptable to you? If everyone who took the pill felt drowsy the next day, you probably wouldn't want to take it. But if only 1 person in a million who took the drug felt drowsy the next day, most of us would be willing to take the chance. So what are the real numbers?

As we said, these numbers aren't as accessible as they should be. We had to track down the original data, which appeared in the biggest scientific study of Lunesta, published in the medical journal *Sleep*.[1] Information from this study was used by the FDA in deciding whether to approve the drug. (We hope that the FDA will change the rules for writing drug ads to require drug makers to include the statistics on side effects directly in the ad, so consumers aren't forced to track down the original studies.)

It turns out that Lunesta actually has quite a few side effects. In the study, people were given either Lunesta or a placebo. In addition to seeing whether Lunesta helped people sleep better, the scientists conducting the study also paid attention to problems people experienced, such as drowsiness, dry mouth, and nausea; and they investigated whether people taking Lunesta had these problems more often than people taking a placebo.

Comparing the results of taking the drug to the results of taking a placebo is crucial; after all, everyone experiences drowsiness, dry mouth, or nausea at one time or another. The normal background level of all these things is captured by seeing how often they occur in the placebo group. By comparing the Lunesta group with the placebo group, scientists can isolate the effects of Lunesta; that is, they can judge how much more often side effects occurred with Lunesta after the background level is accounted for.

In the study, the scientists listed nine side effects that occurred more often with Lunesta. We'll focus on the six most common problems. Just as we did when looking at benefit, we created a table showing the starting risk of each side effect (the percentage of the placebo group who experienced the side effect) and the modified risk (the percentage of the Lunesta group who experienced the side effect).[2]

Symptom Side Effects (Time frame: over 6 months)	Starting Risk (Placebo group)	Modified Risk (Lunesta group)
Unpleasant taste in the mouth (additional 20% due to drug)	6% 6 in 100	26% 26 in 100
Infections (mostly colds) (additional 9% due to drug)	7% 7 in 100	16% 16 in 100
Dizziness (additional 7% due to drug)	3% 3 in 100	10% 10 in 100
Next-day drowsiness (additional 6% due to drug)	3% 3 in 100	9% 9 in 100
Dry mouth (additional 5% due to drug)	2% 2 in 100	7% 7 in 100
Nausea (additional 5% due to drug)	6% 6 in 100	11% 11 in 100

Our list in the table is not the same as the list in the Lunesta advertisement we showed you earlier. We didn't include headaches, for example, since headaches were equally common in both the Lunesta group and the placebo group (that is, the modified risk of headache was the same as the starting risk). Our table does include some side effects that are missing from the ad: infections (mostly more colds), dry mouth, and nausea. The list in the ad is incomplete because the FDA has only vague rules about which side effects must appear in ads.

But as you know by now, a list of side effects isn't very useful unless you know how often they occur with and without the drug. That's why the table gives you the numbers you need.

What is the most common side effect of Lunesta?

    a. Nausea

    b. Dizziness

    c. Unpleasant taste

Who is more likely to have next-day drowsiness?

    a. People taking a placebo

    b. People taking Lunesta

Is this a big difference in next-day drowsiness?

    a. Yes

    b. No

The answer to the first question is c. According to the table, 26 percent of those who took Lunesta complained of an unpleasant taste in the mouth, compared to only 6 percent of those taking the placebo. Remember that 6 percent reflects the background level of unpleasant taste. So the amount of unpleasant taste caused by Lunesta is the difference between 26 percent and 6 percent—that is, 20 percent. In other words, for every 100 people who take Lunesta, an additional 20 will experience an unpleasant taste because of the drug. Nausea is one of the least common side effects—only an additional 5 percent of the participants experienced nausea because they took Lunesta.

    The answer to the second question is b. The table shows that people who took Lunesta were more likely to have next-day drowsiness than people who took the placebo: 9 percent as opposed to 3 percent. That is, for every 100 people who take Lunesta, an additional 6 will experience next-day drowsiness as a result of taking the drug.

    The third question in the quiz has no right answer. Only you can decide whether you care about this or any of the other side effects. Only you can decide whether the differences are big or small. Without the numbers, of course, you cannot even begin to make these judgments.

    You may have noticed that the table includes only bothersome side effects such as nausea and drowsiness; none of them are life-threatening. That's good news for Lunesta. None of the patients in the study experienced any life-threatening problems.

Unfortunately, many drugs do have life-threatening side effects. (Remember Vioxx, the arthritis drug that was pulled from the market because it raised the risk of heart attack and stroke?)

Let's take a look at a drug with some life-threatening side effects. Consider, for example, this advertisement for Nolvadex. (Although Nolvadex is also used to treat breast cancer, the ad and the following discussion focus only on its value in preventing a first occurrence of breast cancer. Nolvadex is now available only in the generic form called tamoxifen.)

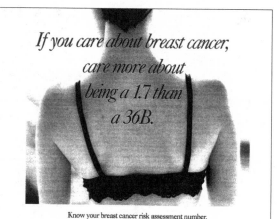

Nolvadex reduces the risk of developing breast cancer (an important patient outcome), but the drug also has rare life-threatening side effects. Here's how the ad describes the side effects.

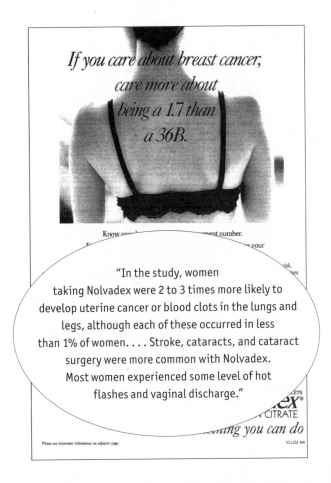

This text in the ad gives you some sense that these side effects are rare, but it doesn't make clear that these problems are life-threatening. And they are: blood clots can kill you, and so can uterine cancer. The following table, which is based on the original Nolvadex study (published in a medical journal, the *Journal of the National Cancer Institute*), categorizes the major side effects of Nolvadex and provides the numbers.[3]

Side Effects (Time frame: over 5 years)	Starting Risk (Placebo group)	Modified Risk (Nolvadex group)
Life-threatening side effects		
Blood clots (in legs or lungs) (additional 0.5% due to drug)	0.5% 5 in 1,000	1.0% 10 in 1,000
Invasive uterine cancer (additional 0.6% due to drug)	0.5% 5 in 1,000	1.1% 11 in 1,000
Symptom side effects		
Hot flashes (additional 12% due to drug)	69% 690 in 1,000	81% 810 in 1,000
Vaginal discharge (additional 20% due to drug)	35% 350 in 1,000	55% 550 in 1,000
Cataracts that needed surgery (additional 0.8% due to drug)	1.5% 15 in 1,000	2.3% 23 in 1,000

As you can see, Nolvadex increases the chance of life-threatening side effects, but fortunately they are still pretty rare. Nolvadex also increases the less serious symptom side effects, but these are pretty common. This situation is typical—symptom side effects are bothersome and common, while life-threatening side effects are serious but rare.

To decide whether a treatment to reduce risk is worth it, you need to think hard about both the size of the benefit and the possible side effects. You have to decide if the possible benefit is worth enough to you to outweigh the chance of side effects. The next chapter shows you how to consider benefits and downsides together.

do the benefits outweigh the downsides? 7

Imagine that you could take a pill that completely protected you against catching a cold. If the pill had no downsides—it was free and convenient and had no symptom or life-threatening side effects—it might sound attractive. But what if the pill caused half the people who took it to have heart attacks? Not so attractive. The point is that focusing solely on a benefit without considering the downsides can be deceptive, even dangerous. The next time you see an ad for a seemingly great new medication or hear a news report touting some medical breakthrough, remember that benefit is only half the story. To judge the value of an intervention, you have to consider potential benefits and downsides together. In the next few pages, we'll look at some examples and do just that. And, as we did before, we won't consider cost or convenience (that's your job) but will instead focus on side effects.

Let's start with Lunesta, the sleeping pill. Earlier we looked at its side effects. The following table, which summarizes findings from the largest and longest-running scientific study of Lunesta, lists the drug's benefits as well as its side effects so that you can get the whole story.[1] It begins by describing some key facts about the study itself: who was studied, how many were studied, and for how long.

788 healthy adults who suffered from insomnia—sleeping less than 6.5 hours per night and/or taking more than 30 minutes to fall asleep—for at least a month were given Lunesta or a placebo nightly for 6 months. Here's what happened.

What Difference Did Lunesta Make?	Starting Risk (Placebo group)	Modified Risk (Lunesta group, 3 mg/night)
Did Lunesta help?		
Lunesta users fell asleep faster (15 minutes faster due to drug)	45 minutes to fall asleep	30 minutes to fall asleep
Lunesta users slept longer (37 minutes longer due to drug)	5 hours, 45 minutes of sleep	6 hours, 22 minutes of sleep
Did Lunesta have side effects?		
Life-threatening side effects No difference between Lunesta and placebo	0% in both groups (none observed in this study)	
Symptom side effects		
Unpleasant taste in the mouth (additional 20% due to drug)	6% 6 in 100	26% 26 in 100
Infections (mostly colds) (additional 9% due to drug)	7% 7 in 100	16% 16 in 100
Dizziness (additional 7% due to drug)	3% 3 in 100	10% 10 in 100
Next-day drowsiness (additional 6% due to drug)	3% 3 in 100	9% 9 in 100
Dry mouth (additional 5% due to drug)	2% 2 in 100	7% 7 in 100
Nausea (additional 5% due to drug)	6% 6 in 100	11% 11 in 100

The table should look familiar—it's just a modification of the tables we constructed in earlier chapters. It shows what people experienced without Lunesta (the starting risk numbers) and with Lunesta (the modified risk numbers). The table is divided into two parts: the top lists the benefits (did Lunesta help?) and the bottom lists the downsides (did Lunesta have side effects?). Providing these two types of information together—and in the same format—makes it possible for you to focus on the real issue at hand: do you believe that the potential benefits are worth the potential side effects?

As you make this judgment, remember to ask one of the key questions we discussed in chapter 4: "Does this risk reduction information reasonably apply to me?" If you are like the people who participated in the study, the table should be a good guide for what to expect if you take the medicine. In this case, being "like the people in the study" means that you're between the ages of 21 and 69 and that you suffer from insomnia (as the study defined it). In addition, you don't have a history of substance abuse, don't use medications or supplements known to affect sleep, and haven't been diagnosed with depression, anxiety, or bipolar disorder.

The less you are like the people in the study, the less you can count on the table to predict your experience. For example, no one knows how the drug works in the elderly or in children—much less whether it is safe. (The FDA has approved it only for adults.) And if you're taking medications that affect sleep, it's hard to know how interactions with those drugs will alter Lunesta's benefits or side effects—other medications taken in conjunction with Lunesta may make Lunesta more or less effective, and they might alter the frequency or intensity of side effects.

Here's how we weighed the benefits against the side effects. To us, the benefits of the drug—falling asleep 15 minutes faster and sleeping 37 minutes longer—seem quite small. In fact, on average, the people in the study who took Lunesta still met the definition of insomnia used in the study even after they took the medication (that is, they still slept less than 6.5 hours and took 30 minutes or more to fall asleep). And we were also struck by the frequency of the bothersome side effects. Overall, we thought that the drug didn't seem to help much and that you would stand a good chance of experiencing some bothersome side effects. We were not impressed.

Remember, however, that what matters is *your* response. How do you weigh the benefits and the side effects? How important are the outcomes to you? You might feel that it's well worth giving the drug a try. You might quickly learn whether it helps or whether it bothers you.

Now let's take another look at Nolvadex (introduced in the previous chapter), the drug used to reduce the chance of developing a first occurrence of breast cancer. The following table provides the information that a woman would need in order to decide whether to take Nolvadex to reduce her breast cancer risk.[2] Looking at benefits and side effects together can help a woman make an informed decision about whether the drug is "worth it" to her.

13,000 women age 35 and older who had never had breast cancer but were considered to be at high risk of getting it were given either Nolvadex or a placebo each day for 5 years. Women were considered to be at high risk if their chance of developing breast cancer over the next 5 years was estimated at 1.7% or higher (an estimate arrived at by using a risk calculator available at www.cancer.gov/bcrisktool). Here's what happened.

What Difference Did Nolvadex Make?	Starting Risk (Placebo group)	Modified Risk (Nolvadex group, 20 mg/day)
Did Nolvadex help?		
Fewer Nolvadex users got invasive breast cancer (1.6% fewer due to drug)	3.3% 33 in 1,000	1.7% 17 in 1,000
No difference in death from breast cancer	About 0.09% in both groups 0.9 in 1,000	
Did Nolvadex have side effects?		
Life-threatening side effects		
Blood clots (in legs or lungs) (additional 0.5% due to drug)	0.5% 5 in 1,000	1.0% 10 in 1,000
Invasive uterine cancer (additional 0.6% due to drug)	0.5% 5 in 1,000	1.1% 11 in 1,000
Symptom side effects		
Hot flashes (additional 12% due to drug)	69% 690 in 1,000	81% 810 in 1,000
Vaginal discharge (additional 20% due to drug)	35% 350 in 1,000	55% 550 in 1,000
Cataracts that needed surgery (additional 0.8% due to drug)	1.5% 15 in 1,000	2.3% 23 in 1,000
Death from all causes combined No difference between Nolvadex and placebo	About 1.2% in both groups 12 in 1,000	

If you are a woman at high risk of getting breast cancer, should you take Nolvadex?

    a. Yes

    b. No

Either answer can be correct. There is no single "right" answer for every individual. We can't tell you the "right" answer, nor can any other physician.

But you can't even begin to make this choice without the numbers. That's the point of this book. With the numbers, you can see that this decision is a close call. But it is much more difficult than the decision whether to take Lunesta. With Lunesta, you can simply try the drug and see whether you experience the benefits or side effects. In the case of Nolvadex, however, the benefits and life-threatening side effects take time to appear (the breast cancers, blood clots, and uterine cancer occurred over 5 years in the study), and they happen to relatively few people. So, even if you don't get breast cancer, you can't really know whether it's because of the drug or just because you had good luck and weren't going to get breast cancer anyway.

For a woman at high risk of breast cancer, deciding whether to take Nolvadex involves a delicate balance between her feelings about the benefit of the drug (lowering the chance of breast cancer) and the side effects, some of which are bothersome and some of which are life-threatening (though rare). The reason we consider this a close call is that it's a situation in which women facing the same risk of breast cancer could reasonably make different choices. On the one hand, you might be a woman who is very worried about developing breast cancer and less worried about the side effects. You might reasonably decide to take the drug. On the other hand, you might be a woman who wonders about the wisdom of starting a medication to address problems that *might* happen in the future (as opposed to taking a medication for a problem you have now). You might be more worried about the problems that the medication can cause and might reasonably decide not to take the drug.

Alternatively, you might choose a middle ground. You might say to yourself, "I'd like to get the benefit of a reduction in breast cancer risk, and I can accept the small increase in the risk of blood clots and uterine cancer. But if the medicine starts making me feel poorly every day, it's not worth it." In this case, you might choose to try the medicine but stop it if you notice any of the common symptom side effects.

Before we leave Nolvadex, let's take another look at the benefit section of the table. The first row indicates that Nolvadex reduced the chance of developing breast cancer. But the second entry states that Nolvadex did *not* reduce the chance of *dying* from breast cancer. How can we explain these two findings? It may be that the drug does in fact decrease the chance of breast cancer death, but the decrease was too small to be picked up in this particular study. (Fortunately, breast cancer deaths were rare among the 13,000 women who participated in the study: a total of 9 died from breast cancer over the 5 years, 6 in the placebo group and 3 in the Nolvadex group—a difference so small that it could have been due to chance, or a fluke.) If this is the case, perhaps a larger, 10-year study might show the small decrease. Another explanation is that the drug may prevent only cancers that are easy to treat and may not prevent the more aggressive forms, so that it really may not reduce the death rate.

No one knows (yet) why Nolvadex did not reduce the chance of breast cancer death. But this does not mean that Nolvadex is useless: avoiding a breast cancer diagnosis and the associated anxiety, surgery, chemotherapy, radiation, and so on is far from trivial. But our point is to emphasize that reducing the risk of getting a disease does not necessarily translate into reducing the risk of dying from the disease. This highlights the importance of knowing where you are on the pyramid of benefit discussed in chapter 5.

An Important Bottom Line: Death from All Causes Combined

There is one other entry in the Nolvadex table that deserves notice: the bottom row, which indicates that the risk of death from all causes combined was the same in the placebo group and the Nolvadex group. The reason you want to know about this statistic has to do with the potential life-threatening side effects of Nolvadex, such as blood clots or uterine cancer. Since these conditions can kill you, it's important to look for any evidence that the drug increases the chance of death from all causes combined. If the drug did increase this chance of death, you'd certainly want to avoid taking it. If it decreased this chance, you'd probably want to take it—if the side effects were not extremely bothersome. In this case, because the drug did not change the chance of death from all causes, you have to make the decision based on the issues we discussed earlier.

The category "death from all causes combined" is a valuable statistic for another reason: there's no ambiguity about it. To understand what we mean, consider the process of counting deaths from specific causes. Sometimes it's hard to know what a person died from. For example, if someone developed severe pneumonia, which triggered a fatal heart attack, did that person die from pneumonia or heart disease? What if a drug caused fewer pneumonia deaths but more heart attack deaths in patients with pneumonia? It is extremely difficult to sort out these ambiguities. That's why death from all causes combined is such a useful measure. There's no way to make a mistake about it: the person is either dead or alive.

Unfortunately, very few medical interventions reduce the chance of dying from all causes combined. The exceptions tend to be drugs like Zocor (discussed in part two), which reduced deaths from all causes combined in a very-high-risk population, people who had already had a heart attack. This is because it reduced the most common cause of death—heart disease—in these patients. Breast cancer does not account for a big proportion of deaths in any age group (see the risk charts in the Extra Help section, pages 128–129); consequently, even eliminating breast cancer completely would make only a small difference in the risk of death from all causes combined. So it wouldn't be "fair" to criticize Nolvadex for not decreasing a woman's overall chance of death. But it's always worth asking how an intervention affects the chance of dying from all causes combined—either as reassurance that life-threatening side effects do not outweigh other benefits or as additional confirmation of the benefit.

Making Decisions

Tables like the ones we've just examined summarize information about medical interventions in a way that clearly conveys the major benefits and side effects and how often they occur. They are helpful not only for consumers who want to make informed decisions about taking medications but also for people facing many other kinds of medical decisions: whether to have an operation, for example, or whether to undergo a screening test such as a PSA test for prostate cancer or a mammogram for breast cancer.

In fact, whenever you face an important medical decision (or other intervention, for that matter), we encourage you to look at such a table. Ask your doctor—or whoever is suggesting the intervention—for one. Or you can construct one yourself. That is, however, easier said than done. Tables like these, and even the data to use in them, are not readily available. But many people are working hard to improve the situation. We are currently collaborating with the U.S. Food and Drug Administration (FDA) to create such tables for prescription drugs. We call them "prescription drug facts boxes," and we hope that they will be available soon.

Meanwhile, to help you find the numbers you need to construct tables, we've listed credible sources of health statistics in the Extra Help section (pages 130–132). All the sources in this list are independent groups that seek to present or summarize the benefits and side effects of medical interventions. It is not intended to be a comprehensive list, but it does include the resources we often use when we are looking for information.

While we are impressed by the quality of information these sources offer, the presentations can vary in how detailed they are and how easy they are to use. The first part of the list consists of sources created primarily for consumers. Unfortunately, these "patient" materials sometimes sacrifice the details you need (that is, the actual numbers) in the name of accessibility. So we encourage you to also explore the second part of the list, which includes sources designed for a physician audience. In these materials, you may find lots of technical terms and acronyms, and you certainly won't find much poetry. But don't be put off; these are great information sources and may be the best places to start looking for good data.

To the extent that you can complete the table with reliable information, you can be confident that you're equipped to make an informed decision. But if you can't fill in large parts of the table—for example, the scientific evidence is not yet available, or there is conflicting evidence—you need to proceed cautiously: you can only guess whether the drug, test, or treatment does more good than harm.

You should recognize, of course, that it makes sense to complete a table like this only when you're facing important decisions with real alternatives. By real alternatives, we mean situations in which you can reasonably choose among different options. Sometimes it's like deciding to put on a life jacket when your ship is sinking: there are no real options, and you just have to act. In the same way, no one would demand to see the scientific evidence that efforts to stop major bleeding after an accident are a good idea. There may also be times when you are facing important choices but are too sick or emotionally overwhelmed to participate in decisions. In this case, friends or family members (who are often looking for ways to be helpful) might be able to seek out information and evaluate the benefits and side effects of various options.

Most of medicine, however, is not about emergencies or situations that don't include real choices. Fortunately, you usually have time to learn about and weigh various options.

The diagram on page 84 summarizes our approach to deciding whether the benefits of a medical intervention outweigh its downsides. Whenever you hear about the benefit of a health intervention, you should ask yourself, "What are the downsides? Is it worth it?"

To answer that question, you must consider whether the action has important side effects, as we've been emphasizing in this chapter, and also assess the cost and inconvenience. If the action is a big deal or has important downsides—that is, it involves a lot of time, pain, or life-threatening side effects—you should insist on an important benefit, one that affects an outcome you really care about. The size of the effect matters, but even small changes in an outcome you care about a lot (like your chance of dying) can be an important benefit. On the other hand, if an intervention changes only a surrogate outcome or an outcome you don't care about so much, the

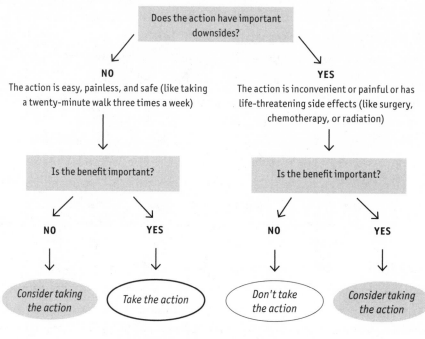

Does the action have important downsides?

NO
The action is easy, painless, and safe (like taking a twenty-minute walk three times a week)

YES
The action is inconvenient or painful or has life-threatening side effects (like surgery, chemotherapy, or radiation)

Is the benefit important?

NO → *Consider taking the action*

YES → *Take the action*

Is the benefit important?

NO → *Don't take the action*

YES → *Consider taking the action*

Definition of an important benefit:
- A small change in the risk of an important outcome that you really care about—like death
- A large change in the risk of a less important outcome

benefit would generally have to be pretty substantial before you would consider the intervention.

If the intervention does *not* have important downsides—it is as easy, painless, and safe as taking a twenty-minute walk three times a week, for example—you may want to do it even if the likely benefit is small (including surrogate outcomes).

For some medical decisions, figuring out whether the benefits outweigh the downsides is easy. But in many cases, it is a balancing act that requires you to carefully judge the importance of the benefits against the downsides.

PART FOUR

developing a healthy skepticism

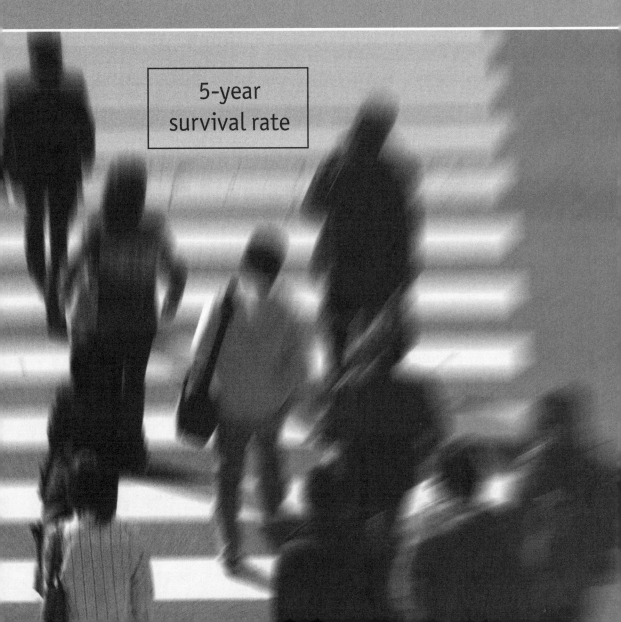

5-year
survival rate

beware of exaggerated importance   8

Health messages—whether advertising, public service announcements, or media reports—often exaggerate their own importance. They may inflate the size of the health problems they present, and they may overstate the benefits of the course of action they promote. When you think about it, it's pretty easy to understand why.

Advertising is all about putting products in the best possible light in order to increase sales and therefore profits. Drug ads are intended to persuade people to take the drugs. As marketing strategy, exaggerating the benefit of a drug and downplaying side effects make sense.

The same logic applies to public service announcements, in which an organization (even with the most altruistic motives) is marketing a behavior: get a flu shot, know your cholesterol level, get screened for breast cancer. Once again, overstatement can help persuade you to do what the organization wants.

Finally, there's no shortage of exaggeration in the media. News reports are especially good vehicles for exaggeration because so many people and organizations stand to gain financially and professionally from being associated with exciting news. Strongly favorable news coverage spurs sales for drug and device manufacturers, which in turn rewards their investors. Being associated with widely reported "breakthroughs" advances the careers of scientists and is a plus for their sponsors. Good publicity helps health care providers sign up patients and bolsters the causes of patient advocacy groups by attracting donors. Finally, media outlets themselves benefit from attention-getting news coverage: compelling stories sell papers and help journalists get their work on page one. As these forces converge, a self-reinforcing cycle of exaggeration is probably inevitable.

So what can you do? Our advice is to be a healthy skeptic. That doesn't mean you have to be a cynic, simply disbelieving all the health messages you hear. Instead, it means approaching messages critically: looking out for—and seeing through—common tactics used to exaggerate the importance of health problems or actions you can take to address them. These tactics include emphasizing unimportant outcomes, avoiding numbers, or presenting statistics in ways that make them seem more important than they really are.

These two basic steps, which we've emphasized throughout the book, will help you to think clearly and critically about a health message:

Step 1. Be clear that the outcome matters to you. To begin deciphering a health message, you need to determine which outcome is being considered. If you don't care about that outcome, then it makes no sense to act on—or think about acting on—the message. For example, you may hear that millions of Americans have prehypertension—that is, their blood pressure is at the high end of the range considered normal. Should you worry about whether you have prehypertension or take some kind of treatment for it? We would say no unless you are shown convincing evidence that this condition matters—that the people with prehypertension do worse in some tangible way or do better if treated.

Step 2. Get the numbers. The second step is to look critically at all the alarming numbers or dramatic stories that are being used to grab your attention. Consider the following news story leads:

> "Mrs. Jones (shown here with her three young children) was diagnosed with liver cancer in 2003. She took drug X, and her cancer melted away."

> "Liver cancer will strike almost 19,000 people this year."

> "A new study has found that drug Y reduces deaths from liver cancer by 67 percent!"

> "A new study has found that drug Z reduces liver cancer deaths from 3 in 100,000 to 1 in 100,000."

Which stories grab your attention? Everybody responds to a compelling anecdote (the first lead). For most of us, an ounce of emotional content is worth a pound of data.

Big numbers also catch your attention (the second lead), as do large relative changes like the 67 percent relative change in liver cancer deaths (the third lead). This is a common tactic, which can leave you with an exaggerated sense of how well treatment works.

And, of course, a dry report of the starting and modified risks (the fourth lead) is both less impressive than the big numbers and much less compelling than the story about a person with young children whose life was "saved" by an experimental drug.

But, as you know by now, you need the data. Without the numbers, it's hard to tell how big the risk really is, how big the benefit might be, or how much it matters to you. The only way to assess the importance of anecdotes ("Smith says he lowered his cholesterol by eating garlic") and *qualitative claims* ("mammograms save lives" or "statins reduce heart disease") is to examine *quantitative data*—specifically, the frequency of an outcome among people who receive or do not receive a treatment (the starting and modified risks).

Our advice can really be summarized in six words: know the outcome; get the numbers! You apply this principle regularly in daily life. How you react to news that taxes are increasing, rents in your building are going up, or salaries in your firm will rise depends entirely on the size of the increase. When it comes to money, it's hard to imagine anyone who would hear the phrase "going up" and not want to know what the real numbers are. But, surprisingly, many people don't demand the same kind of complete information when they hear health messages. We hope that you will.

A Special Case of Exaggerated Numbers: Survival Statistics

If there were a hall of fame for exaggeration, survival statistics would get a lifetime achievement award. Survival statistics are widely used. Unfortunately, they are also widely misused and easily misunderstood, even when you know the starting and modified risks. Because these statistics come up so often in cancer screening, we'd like to explain how they work.

Cancer screening means testing people who have no symptoms to look for hidden, early evidence of cancer. The assumption is that if you find cancer in very early stages, when a tumor is small, it is less likely to have spread to other parts of the body and is more likely to be curable.

There are many tests that can be used for screening, including mammography for breast cancer, colonoscopy for colon cancer, and PSA testing for prostate cancer. You should be clear that how a test gets used determines whether it is a screening test. When a woman who has no signs or symptoms of breast cancer goes for her annual mammogram, she is getting a screening test. But when a woman feels a lump in her breast and gets a mammogram, she is not getting a screening test—she is getting a diagnostic test in response to a symptom.

You'll often hear survival statistics quoted to demonstrate the value of screening. The most common statistic used is a 5-year survival rate. There's nothing special about a span of 5 years. Survival statistics can be calculated for any time period. The lung and prostate cancer examples we'll discuss in the next pages use both 5- and 10-year survival statistics. For either time frame, the issues that you need to understand are identical.

Here's a typical example of how survival statistics are misused. This example is an excerpt from a story published in the *Los Angeles Times* in 2006:[1]

Study Calls for Routine CT Scans for Smokers

The use of advanced CT imaging to detect lung tumors in their still-treatable early stages greatly increases survival rates, and smokers should be routinely screened just as women are for breast cancer, according to a report today in the *New England Journal of Medicine*.

Imaging yielded an estimated 10-year survival rate of more than 90%, researchers said. Currently, about 5% of the 174,000 lung cancer patients diagnosed each year survive for 10 years. . . .

"This is compelling evidence that you can use CT screening to find lung cancer . . . and when you find it early and take it out early, you can cure a high percentage of patients," said Dr. Claudia I. Henschke of Cornell University's Weill Medical College in New York City, who led the study.

These results sound almost miraculous: CT scans for smokers seem to change the 10-year survival rate for lung cancer patients from 5 percent to over 90 percent. Does this prove that CT screening works? The short answer is no. To understand why not, you have to consider exactly how a 10-year survival rate is calculated. It is a fraction that, in this case, tells you what proportion of a group of people diagnosed with lung cancer is still alive 10 years later. Imagine 1,000 people diagnosed with lung cancer 10 years ago. If 50 are alive today, the 10-year survival rate is 50 / 1,000, or 5 percent. If 900 are alive today, the 10-year survival rate is 900 / 1,000, or 90 percent. Yet even if CT screening raised the 10-year survival rate to 90 percent, it is entirely possible that none of these patients will get an extra day of life.

The best way to understand this is to work through two thought experiments. First, consider a group of people with lung cancer who will all die at age 70. If they first receive the diagnosis when they are 67, their 10-year survival rate is 0 percent. (Do you see why? If they all die at age 70, none will be alive 10 years later.) But if these same people had received CT scans that found their cancer before they had symptoms, they would have been diagnosed earlier—at, say, age 57—and their 10-year survival rate would have been 100 percent. Yet death would still come at age 70. Earlier diagnosis *always* increases survival rates, but it doesn't necessarily mean that death is postponed. This diagram helps you review how this happens.

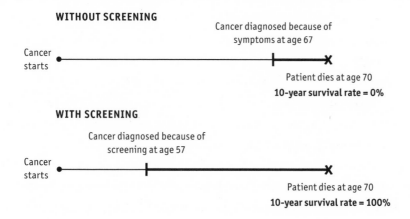

In other words, making the diagnosis earlier does not in itself mean that you delay death. It may simply mean that you know about the cancer for a longer time.

Comparing survival rates when people are diagnosed with a disease in different ways—for instance, based on a CT scan versus based on symptoms—is always misleading. That's because the CT scans are great at finding early, hidden cancers, and survival rates always go up when diagnoses are made in early stages.

A second thought experiment helps to explain why CT scans, which find so many minute tumors, can inflate survival rates even if no lives are saved. It turns out that some forms of cancer look like cancer under the microscope but do not behave the way we might expect cancer to—that is, they do not develop into a relentlessly progressive, deadly disease. These nonprogressive cancers grow so slowly that they never cause symptoms, nor do they affect how long a person lives. Consequently, the only way we can diagnose these nonprogressive tumors is by screening.

Prostate cancer provides the most familiar example. We can find microscopic evidence of prostate cancer in around half of 60-year-old men if we look hard enough. Yet only 3 in 1,000 will die from prostate cancer over the next 10 years. How can this be? Because prostate cancer isn't just one disease: it's a spectrum of disorders. Some forms of prostate cancer grow very rapidly and kill the men who have them. Some grow so slowly that, even without treatment, men die of something else before the cancer causes symptoms. And other forms look like cancer under the microscope but never grow at all or may regress spontaneously. While this phenomenon is best understood in prostate cancer, it probably occurs in all cancers.

Now imagine a city in which 1,000 people are found to have lung cancer following evaluation for cough and weight loss (symptoms of lung cancer). At 10 years after diagnosis, 50 are alive and 950 have died, which equals a 10-year survival rate of 5 percent. Now let's start again—but this time imagine that everyone in the city is screened with CT scans. In this scenario, 5,000 are given a cancer diagnosis: the 1,000 who had symptoms, plus 4,000 others who actually have nonprogressive cancers. These 4,000 would not die from lung cancer in 10 years. Consequently, the 10-year survival rate for lung cancer in the city would increase dramatically—to 81 percent—because these healthy people would appear in both parts of the fraction: 4,050 / 5,000. But what has really changed? Some people were unnecessarily told that they had cancer (and may have undergone harmful therapy), but the same number of people (950) still died. We have sketched out this scenario in the following diagram.

WITHOUT SCREENING

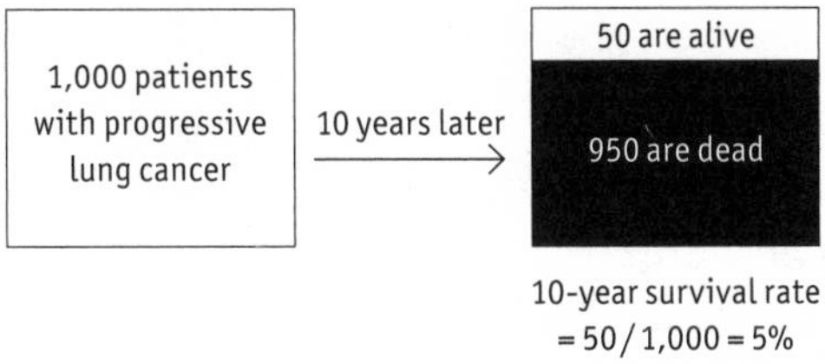

1,000 patients with progressive lung cancer

10 years later →

50 are alive

950 are dead

10-year survival rate = 50 / 1,000 = 5%

WITH SCREENING

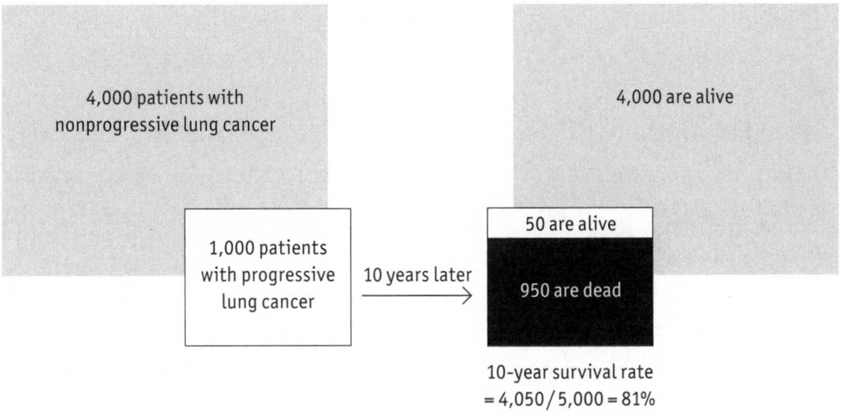

4,000 patients with nonprogressive lung cancer

4,000 are alive

1,000 patients with progressive lung cancer

10 years later →

50 are alive

950 are dead

10-year survival rate = 4,050 / 5,000 = 81%

The idea that screening can increase survival rates without actually saving lives is not just a theory. It was confirmed in a randomized trial of regular chest X-ray screening at the Mayo Clinic involving more than 9,000 male smokers.[2] In that trial, 5-year survival rates were almost two times higher for those who had been screened than for those who had not been screened (35 percent versus 19 percent), but death rates were the same in the two groups. In fact, the death rate was slightly higher in the screened group. Consequently, doctors do not recommend lung cancer screening with chest X-rays.

Survival statistics and death statistics sound like two ways of talking about the same thing. But they are not flip sides of the same coin. To understand how this works, it helps to look at how these kinds of statistics are calculated.

Let's start with survival statistics. As an example, let's calculate the 5-year survival rate for a particular type of cancer (we'll call it cancer X). As explained earlier, the 5-year survival rate for a group of patients diagnosed with cancer X is the number of people in the group who are alive 5 years after their cancer diagnosis, divided by the number originally diagnosed. Here's the formula:

$$\text{5-year survival rate} = \frac{\text{number of patients alive 5 years after diagnosis}}{\substack{\text{number of patients originally} \\ \text{diagnosed with cancer X}}}$$

Now let's calculate a death statistic, which typically refers to a 1-year time frame (you can think of it as presenting a 1-year risk of death). For example, the death rate (or *mortality rate,* as researchers call it) for cancer X is the number of people in a group who die from that cancer over 1 year, divided by the number of people in the group. Here's the formula:

$$\text{Annual death rate} = \text{1-year risk of death}$$

$$= \frac{\text{number of people who died from cancer X over 1 year}}{\text{all people in the group}}$$

The key thing to notice is how the denominator (the bottom number in the fraction) for survival statistics differs from the denominator for death statistics. For survival rates, the denominator is the number of patients diagnosed with the illness; for death rates, it is all the people in a group (which could be, for instance, the population of a country, an age group, or some other defined group).

Survival statistics are always distorted by screening. As you saw in the last two illustrations (pages 91 and 93), survival statistics can go up even when the same number of people die. So survival statistics cannot tell you whether fewer people are dying from cancer.

In contrast, death rates can tell you what is really happening. If finding early cancer delays death, the annual death rate indeed goes down, since fewer people are dying in that year. But if screening is finding only more nonprogressive cancer, the death rate doesn't change.

But comparing survival rates and death rates is like comparing apples and oranges. In fact, when you look at our best national cancer data, you will find no relationship between improved 5-year survival rates and death rates over time.[3] For example, the 5-year survival rate for melanoma, the most deadly form of skin cancer, has improved from 49 percent in 1950 to 92 percent in the most recent data available. But death rates have actually gone up during this same period, from 1 death in 100,000 to almost 3 deaths in 100,000.[4]

So when you hear about changes in survival rates among people who have been screened for a disease, you cannot automatically assume that these changes reflect fewer deaths from the disease. Such changes could simply mean that we are diagnosing more early cases of disease but not delaying death, or that we are finding more nonprogressive disease. In other words, improved survival rates among people who have been screened for a disease provide no evidence that screening works to reduce deaths. The only way to know whether screening works is to show that death rates are lower in the screened group. Screening may well reduce deaths from a disease, but survival statistics are never a good guide to whether this is happening.

When used for the right purpose, however, survival statistics can be a good guide. The Learn More box on the next page shows you how survival statistics can be used appropriately to estimate your prognosis (your chance of surviving for a fixed period of time with a particular disease) and to judge the benefit of a treatment.

Learn More

When Survival Statistics Are Not Misleading

Although survival statistics are misleading in assessing the value of screening, they are not misleading when used for two other purposes: as a prognosis for an individual patient and as an outcome in a randomized trial.

When you are diagnosed with a serious illness, survival statistics are used to estimate your prognosis—your chance of surviving for a fixed period of time. As we've discussed throughout the book, these statistics are most relevant to you when they are based on people like you, people who are similar in age and gender and who have similar health conditions.

Another characteristic that determines your prognosis is the stage of the disease (how advanced it is). The most useful survival statistics are those generated for people whose illness is at the same stage as yours. For example, in early-stage cancer, the cancer may be localized to one organ. By the intermediate stage, it may have spread to the tissue around the organ. Late-stage cancer means that it has spread to other parts of the body. The federal government has created a great source of stage-specific survival statistics for cancer, known as SEER (Surveillance, Epidemiology, and End Results).[5]

Survival statistics are also a meaningful way to judge the benefit of a treatment—for example, does a new cancer drug prolong life? To answer this question, researchers conduct randomized trials comparing a group of people taking the new drug to a control group of people who are not taking it. The results of these trials yield the starting and modified risks (similar to the risks we calculated for Zocor in chapter 4). The outcome is often expressed as a 5-year survival statistic: the fraction of people in each group who survive for 5 years divided by the number of people in that group.

Consider this example: drug X is used to treat people diagnosed with stage 1 pancreatic cancer. In a randomized trial, people age 50 to 75 years with stage 1 pancreatic cancer were randomly assigned to take either drug X or the standard drug (the control group). Drug X improved survival.

Starting risk = 5-year survival rate in the control group = 20%
Modified risk = 5-year survival rate in the drug X group = 30%

Because randomization creates groups that should be similar in every way (including how they were diagnosed), comparing these starting and modified survival statistics provides a good measure of how well treatment works.

This discussion about survival rates and death rates may seem a little counterintuitive. To help make sure you understand the ideas we've covered, take a look at the following chart, which appeared in a 1990 brochure sent to patients by the M. D. Anderson Cancer Center, a major academic medical center in Texas.

"As national mortality rates fluctuated between 1960 and 1990, five-year survival rates for prostate cancer among our patients continued to improve."

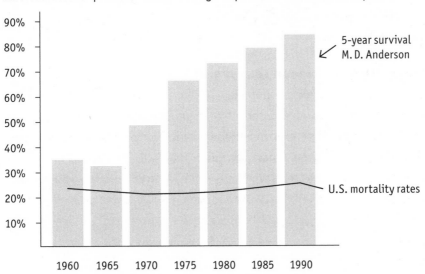

The correct answer to the first question is c. It turns out that U.S. survival rates for prostate cancer—not just the survival rates for M. D. Anderson's patients—also went up dramatically during this period, from about 40 percent in 1960 to 90 percent in 1990. This increase in 5-year survival reflects the growth of prostate cancer screening with the PSA blood test. In fact, the average U.S. 5-year survival rate of 90 percent was, ironically, higher than the survival rate at M. D. Anderson. To judge whether fewer people are dying of prostate cancer, death rates are the right measure to use. Unfortunately, this line in the chart looks pretty flat—suggesting that deaths from prostate cancer in the United States did not change much over this time. Comparing the 5-year survival rates of M. D. Anderson's patients with overall U.S. mortality rates is nonsense.

The correct answer to the Extra Credit question is c, 70 percent. Here's how we did the calculations. First, we wrote out the fraction for the 5-year survival rate of 40 percent:

$$\frac{400 \text{ patients with cancer X alive 5 years after diagnosis}}{1,000 \text{ patients originally diagnosed with cancer X}} = 40\%$$

Then we added the 1,000 people with nonprogressive cancer to both the numerator and the denominator:

$$\frac{\begin{array}{c}400 \text{ patients with cancer X} + 1,000 \text{ patients with} \\ \text{nonprogressive cancer X alive 5 years after diagnosis}\end{array}}{\begin{array}{c}1,000 \text{ patients diagnosed with cancer X} + \\ 1,000 \text{ diagnosed with nonprogressive cancer X}\end{array}} = \frac{1,400}{2,000} = 70\%$$

Although this example may be a little difficult to follow at first, it allows you to see for yourself how dramatically 5-year survival rates can change when nonprogressive cancers are diagnosed—although no one has lived any longer.

beware of exaggerated certainty 9

Of course, the numbers you see in health messages are not the whole story. We'd now like to add another bit of advice: once you have the numbers, ask yourself whether or not you should believe them. Unfortunately, many statistics should not be accepted at face value, because they convey a sense of exaggerated certainty. There are at least two reasons why reported research findings might not be right: much research is based on weak science, and many results are disseminated too early.

What Kind of Science Is Behind the Numbers?

The first question to ask is, "Is there any science behind the numbers?" Ideally, there would be. But sometimes there isn't. The second question is, "How good is the science?" Some research makes only a weak case for the message; other studies make a strong case. In this section, we'll help you think about how compelling the case is.

For example, treatments that have been shown to fight illnesses in test tubes don't necessarily make you better. And treatments that work in animals often don't have the same results in humans. This doesn't mean that basic science research is not important—indeed, it is fundamental. But it's important to be skeptical about treatments that have been proven only in animal or lab studies, since they may not turn out to be relevant for people. Even when we focus on the most promising animal studies, only about one-third of treatments proven helpful in animals have turned out to be helpful in people.[1] The following diagram illustrates a spectrum of believability for research findings; we put test tube and animal studies lowest on our believability scale because these findings often do not translate into improved human health.

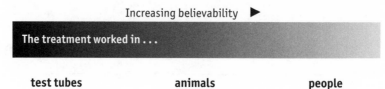

Increasing believability ▶

The treatment worked in . . .

test tubes   animals   people

And not all human research studies are equally compelling, either. In an *observational uncontrolled study,* researchers simply watch what happens to a series of people in one group. For example, everyone gets drug X, and the researchers record how many people get better. But there's a big problem with these studies: you can't know what would have happened *without* drug X —maybe more people would have gotten better! Whenever you hear the results of a study about how well an intervention works, ask whether the study included a *control group* (a group of people who did not undergo the intervention). Without a control group, it's impossible to know whether the intervention really accounts for the study findings. Remind yourself that, no matter how dramatically the findings from an uncontrolled study are described, they are not particularly believable.

Stronger scientific evidence comes from *controlled studies,* in which researchers watch what happens to different groups of people. The most basic kinds of controlled studies involve observational research, in which the researchers merely record what happens to people in different situations, without intervening. Cohort and case-control studies are perhaps the best-known types of *observational controlled research.* Such research first linked cigarette smoking to lung cancer, and high cholesterol to heart disease. This is the only way to study dangerous exposures. But these kinds of studies have important problems. Although they can show that an intervention is *associated* with a particular outcome, they cannot by themselves prove that the intervention *causes* the outcome. It's always possible that other factors not accounted for in the research are causing the outcome.

For example, researchers might believe that eating string beans prevents heart attacks. To test this hypothesis, they compare people who eat a lot of string beans with people who never eat string beans to see which group has more heart attacks. Of course, these groups of people may be very different in lots of ways besides eating string beans. For instance, let's say that people who choose to eat string beans might be more likely to be vegetarians, to eat a Mediterranean diet, and to exercise. So if the string bean eaters "do better" than the others, it might not be because of the string beans.

An actual example involves the long-held belief that most women should take estrogen after menopause. That idea, only recently discredited, also came from observational research. The observation—drawn from more than forty studies involving hundreds of thousands of women—was that women who took estrogen supplements had less heart disease. But it turned out that estrogen was not the reason for decreased heart disease. Instead, women taking estrogen tended to be healthier and wealthier. Their health and wealth—not their estrogen supplements—were responsible for the lower risk of heart disease.

Whenever you hear about the results of observational controlled studies, we suggest being cautious about concluding that the lifestyle factor, environmental exposure, or drug being studied (like eating string beans or taking estrogen) actually causes the outcome (like heart disease). In these types of studies, you simply cannot rule out the possibility that another characteristic of the participants in fact caused the difference—and that the original conclusion may therefore be wrong. Although we are stuck with observational studies when we research harmful exposures such as smoking, this is fortunately not the case for learning the benefit of an intervention.

The only way to reliably tell if the intervention causes the outcome is to conduct a true experiment—a randomized trial. In a *randomized controlled trial,* researchers construct two groups that are similar in every way except one: whether or not they get the intervention being studied. Patients are assigned randomly (by chance) to one of the groups. It is then reasonable to assume that any differences observed in the trial must have been caused by the intervention (since it was the only difference between the groups). In the case of the assumed connection between estrogen and heart disease, such a study showed that the long-held beliefs were wrong.

In general, you can have the most faith in statistics resulting from large, randomized, controlled trials. Having a large number of study participants is important to make sure that the findings are not the result of chance and to get a precise estimate of the difference between the starting and modified risks. It's sometimes even possible to combine the results of multiple randomized trials to get even more reliable and precise results, using an approach called meta-analysis. This diagram summarizes the believability of the results of different study designs.

Increasing believability ▶

The treatment worked in . . .			
Observational Studies		**Experiments**	
Series of patients with no comparison group	Series of patients with comparison group	Single randomized trial	Multiple randomized trials

But even when results come from a randomized trial, they aren't necessarily right. The results of randomized trials can also be misleading—particularly if the trial was small (for example, with fewer than thirty participants) or lasted only a short time (like a few months). And, as we noted earlier, the benefit of any treatment should be weighed against its side effects or other downsides, such as inconvenience or cost—and these may not have been measured in the randomized trial.

Unfortunately, it's not always possible to conduct a randomized trial. This is certainly the case for studying harmful exposures such as smoking. Because it's unethical to deliberately expose people to harm, the best we can do in such cases is an observational study. And sometimes even when it is ethical to conduct a randomized trial, it might not be feasible. For example, it's extremely unlikely that we could get people to agree to be randomly assigned to eat either only fast food or only organic food every day for a year (or that they would actually adhere to the diet). Again, in such cases, scientists have to rely on observational studies.

But when new interventions are proposed, it is critical to conduct randomized trials before these new strategies are introduced into widespread

Learn More

About This Book

Randomized trials are conducted not only to evaluate drugs—they can also test all sorts of interventions. We actually tested how an early draft of this book affected readers' ability to understand messages about risk (and risk reduction).

We conducted two randomized trials to see how well the book performed in two distinct populations. The first trial included 334 people who attended a public lecture series at Dartmouth Medical School. This lecture series is especially popular with retirees in the community. The second trial included 221 veterans and their families recruited from the waiting areas in the medical clinic at our local Veterans Administration Hospital, where we see patients. The people attending the lecture series tend to be much more affluent and to have more formal education than the people from the VA.

Other than these differences among the participants, the trials were identical. People were randomly assigned to read either our book or a general education book of about the same length and reading level that included no training in understanding risk. This second book served as our "placebo." Everyone was asked to answer an eighteen-question test, which asked them to interpret real-world health statistics in drug advertisements and news stories.[2]

The results—published in the *Annals of Internal Medicine*— were very gratifying for us.[3] In both trials, the book proved to be effective (and safe). Here's what we found:

	Starting Risk (With "placebo" book)	Modified Risk (With our book)
Did our book help?		
Lecture series trial		
Got a passing grade on test	56%	74%
Got an A on test	7%	26%
VA trial		
Got a passing grade on test	26%	44%
Got an A on test	2%	10%
Did our book have side effects?	None reported	

This means this book is clinically proven to be effective!

use.[4] Doctors prescribed estrogen to millions of women for many years until randomized trials showed that intuition and dozens of observational studies were wrong.

Is It Too Early?

The other reason why even the most exciting findings might be wrong is that they are premature. Regardless of the study design—whether observational, randomized, or another type—you should *always* be extremely cautious about preliminary findings. Many of the most impressive breakthroughs reported in the media are first announced at meetings of medical or scientific associations. But these results are often preliminary—the study may not even be finished, and sometimes the results have not yet been vetted by outside experts, a process known as *peer review*. Some of the results presented at such meetings may never be published in professional medical journals because of concerns about whether the findings are really valid. Or, if the findings are published, they may change substantially, perhaps even contradicting the results first reported.[5] In other words, such reports sometimes turn out to be wrong. So we recommend a very high level of skepticism when the media trumpets the results of unpublished research presented at professional meetings.

Other results are too early because they are based on short-term studies. It takes time to verify and confirm research results. The problems that arise with newly approved prescription drugs are an all too common example. In the studies required for approval by the U.S. Food and Drug Administration (FDA), researchers typically test drugs in relatively small groups of people for a relatively short time. Consequently, rare or long-term side effects will not be seen until after approval, when the drug goes on the market and millions of people use it for long periods. This is why you often hear about the FDA either removing a drug from the market or putting a "black box warning" on it to let people know about a new side effect that has turned up.

In general, it's a good idea to be wary of new drugs. We would even go so far as to advise avoiding them unless there is no good alternative. Most serious problems with new drugs emerge within 5 years of FDA approval, so it might be wise to stick with drugs that have been around for at least 5 years rather than going with a new one.[6] With drugs, it's dangerous to assume that newer means better. You should be skeptical of the claim that newer drugs must be better drugs.

You'll find a lot of exaggerated certainty out there. Look out for "strong" conclusions based on weak science. Pay the most attention to research results that have been independently reviewed by experts and are published in reputable medical journals. Approach preliminary work skeptically. And be cautious about new drugs and treatments until they have established a track record for safety and effectiveness.

who's behind the numbers? 10

The last issue we want to raise also has to do with whether to believe the numbers. In addition to being aware of the underlying science, as the previous chapter discussed, it's also important to be aware of the people who produce the numbers. Ideally, researchers do not have a vested interest in how their study turns out; they are concerned only that the research was performed correctly. In reality, however, researchers may stand to benefit personally or professionally if the test or treatment being studied works well—in other words, they may have a conflict of interest.

The most blatant conflicts of interest involve money. The most obvious example is the direct involvement of industry in research. Pharmaceutical companies and device manufacturers need to sell their products. Research showing that the products work well is crucial, as is generating excitement about the products among physicians and the public. Financial conflicts of interest can influence every phase of the process, from the design of the research through its dissemination (as summarized in the table on page 110). A growing literature suggests that, unfortunately, these conflicts of interest are common and influential.[1]

Studies can be designed to stack the deck in favor of a company's product. Outcome measures can be crafted to show impressive differences that distract everyone from asking fundamental questions, such as "Does the finding really matter?" There can be selective publication of only the most favorable studies and the most favorable findings within studies. And, after publication, results can be spun for public consumption by launching public relations and ad campaigns that use the compelling presentation tactics

Phase of Research or Dissemination	Tactic to Generate Exaggerated Result
Study design	Conducting studies that stack the deck in favor of the product • by comparing it to a placebo rather than to another drug that treats the same problem, because it is much easier to look better than nothing (the placebo) than to look better than a proven drug • by comparing it to the "weakest" drug that treats the same problem (for example, choosing the least effective drug for comparison, or using the other drug at a low dose) • by measuring less important surrogate outcomes, where it is easier and faster to show a difference
Publication of scientific results	Selectively publishing only the studies with the most favorable results (rather than all studies) Selectively reporting only favorable outcomes in medical journal articles or in prescription drug labels (or purposely omitting worrisome outcomes)
"Spinning" the results to the public	Using unrepresentative patient anecdotes, citing a "miracle cure" rather than the typical effect among patients Making strong statements about how impressive the results are (but failing to provide any numbers) Using the biggest numbers possible to describe how many people have the problem or how big the benefit is (typically by providing only the relative change in outcomes) Exaggerating what is good and minimizing what is bad about the product
Public campaigns to promote use of the intervention	Scaring people into adopting the intervention, by highlighting the great danger of the problem or the great danger of failing to take action Shaming people into adopting the intervention, by equating its use with being a socially responsible person

outlined in chapter 9. In addition, disease advocacy groups or paid research consultants can be mobilized to use the same tactics to reach the public directly and through the news media.

Of course, money can also influence physicians directly. For example, a doctor who invents and patents a new test for heart disease (or owns stock in the company that holds the patent) can earn a lot more money if the test appears to work really well. So can the researchers and investors involved with the growing number of companies that offer genetic testing services. Papers touting the association of specific genes with increased risk of diseases as diverse as prostate cancer and restless legs syndrome can mean big money when published in high-profile journals—even if no one knows what, if anything, to do based on the results.

Financial conflicts of interest have been the focus of great attention in the past few years, and many medical journals have begun to require that researchers disclose potential conflicts when they publish their work. To be honest, it's not clear how well this is working. Most journals just don't have the resources to verify disclosures for accuracy and instead must rely on the honesty of the researchers.

But there are other, less blatant forces that can also create a conflict of interest. We understand these forces because we are researchers too. Many researchers desire prestige and publicity, both of which help us advance in the academic world. Most researchers strongly believe that what they're studying does, in fact, work—understandably, that belief motivates us to do the research in the first place and to see it through. These forces lead to what we call professional conflicts of interest. All of us have them to various degrees.

While financial conflicts of interest are the most powerful, both types of conflict can affect the quality of scientists' work. In the most extreme cases, research has actually been faked. A recent, infamous example involved bone marrow transplants as a treatment for breast cancer patients.[2] Researchers conducting a randomized controlled trial in South Africa reported amazing results: 51 percent of women who received bone marrow transplants had no evidence of tumor after treatment, compared to only 4 percent of those who received standard treatment. Unfortunately, the researchers had lied, and the results were fiction. Two randomized trials subsequently showed that bone marrow transplantation—which has serious side effects—did not help breast cancer patients. Luckily, such deception is pretty rare. The much more common problem is that conflicts of interest lead researchers to exaggerate the importance of their findings.

Researchers occasionally act more like advocates than scientists, which can lead them to "spin" their results. As outlined in the table on page 110, they may make extreme overstatements to the media about the importance of their work, or they may use anecdotes irresponsibly—telling the story of the one patient who experienced a "miracle cure" and ignoring the less impressive effects on more typical patients. They sometimes make strong assertions about how important their results are (typically without providing actual numbers), or they endeavor to present the biggest numbers possible. And they often exaggerate what is good (information that is favorable to their test or treatment) and minimize what is bad (information that is unfavorable, such as side effects).

In addition, there are well-meaning organizations—patient advocacy groups and public health agencies—who may use these same tactics to promote their particular causes.[3] They strongly believe that they have identified problems that really matter and offer solutions that really work. They argue that the main obstacle they face is getting people to listen and to do the right thing—that is, to follow their advice and eat less fat, get more flu shots, undergo screening for cancer, and so on. Unfortunately, they sometimes resort to fear and shame to achieve these ends. For example, the March of Dimes ran a campaign that equated an expectant mother who does not take folate (a vitamin supplement that reduces the chance of rare neural tube defects from about 2 in 1,000 births to about 1 in 1,000) with a mother who lets her baby crawl into oncoming traffic. And slogans such as "If you haven't had a recent mammogram, you may need more than your breasts examined" are pretty clear: no sane woman would choose to forgo screening.

Regardless of who is behind exaggeration—or what their motivation is—a host of other individuals and organizations are eager to amplify it, including university public relations machines, advocacy groups, and, of course, the news media.

So it's important to consider whether the people behind the numbers benefit from the health messages you receive. Whenever you hear someone touting a new test or treatment, it's a good idea to ask whether the researcher or the organization that paid for the work stands to benefit financially (or otherwise) from its success. Increasingly, you can find answers about who is funding research. Disclosure information is now routinely available in medical journal articles and in the article index in the U.S. National Library of Medicine.[4] The federal government's registry of clinical trials[5] also provides funding information. Discovering the affiliations of organizations or professional experts quoted in the news can be tricky. Journalists sometimes report this information in news stories, but not reliably. One useful source is the Integrity in Science Project, a database sponsored by the Center for Science in the Public Interest, which allows you to search for corporate conflicts of interest among scientists and nonprofit organizations.[6]

Be wary of information from sources that have important interests—besides your health—in promoting a new treatment or product. This doesn't mean that you should dismiss what they have to say out of hand. It just makes it more imperative that you get all the relevant numbers. Then you can decide for yourself whether the news is too good to be true.

We hope this book will help you approach health messages critically—not with cynicism, but with healthy skepticism. This means not accepting claims at face value, because they come from a prestigious source or because it feels like everyone else accepts them. It is worth reexamining a diagram that we presented earlier in the book:

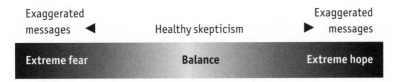

Healthy skepticism helps you push back against unfounded and exaggerated claims and avoid unnecessary fear and false hope. It takes discipline to look beyond claims—to find out the numbers, to evaluate the science they are based on, and to learn who is behind the claims. But that's what you have to do—and what you are now ready to do—to really know your chances.

extra help

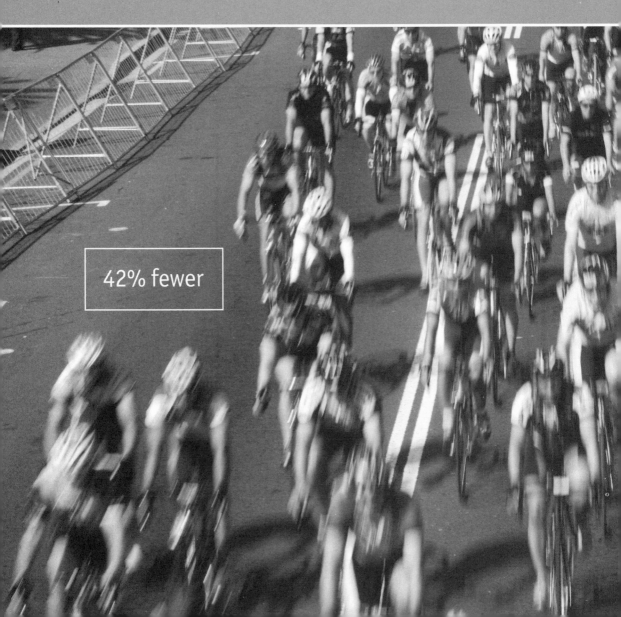

42% fewer

QUICK SUMMARY

Questions to Ask When Interpreting Risk

Risk of what?   Understand what the outcome is (getting a disease, dying from a disease, developing a symptom), and consider how bad it is.

How big is the risk?   Find out your chance of experiencing the outcome. If you hear about the number of people who experience an outcome, always ask, "Out of how many?" You need to know how many people could have experienced the outcome in order to calculate your own chance. Also ask, "What is the time frame?" Is the time frame for the risk the next year, the next 10 years, or a lifetime?

Because there are many ways to express the same risk, it's useful to put information in a consistent format. Our choice would be "___ out of 1,000 people over 10 years."

To get the full picture, we also suggest that you reframe the risk: for example, if 5 out of 1,000 people die over 10 years, it is also true that 995 out of 1,000 will *not* die.

Does the risk information reasonably apply to me?   Determine whether the message is based on studies of people like you (people of your age and sex, people whose health is like yours).

How does this risk compare with other risks?   Get some perspective by asking about other risks you face so that you can develop a sense of just how big (or small) this particular risk really is.

Questions to Ask When Interpreting Risk Reduction

Reduced risk of what?   Understand what outcome is being changed, and decide how much you care about it. Is it something you directly experience, such as symptoms or death (a patient outcome)? Or is it just a blood test or X-ray result (a surrogate outcome)?

Be most skeptical about interventions that have been shown to improve only surrogate outcomes, because changes in surrogate outcomes do not reliably translate into feeling better or living longer. The less you care about the outcome, the less important it is to think about the size of the benefit.

How big is the risk reduction?   Find out your chance of experiencing the outcome if you don't take an action (such as taking a medication or changing your lifestyle) and your chance if you do take the action. In other words, know your modified and starting risks. This is especially important if you hear a message such as "drug X lowers your risk by 42 percent." Always ask, "Lower than what?" Unless you know your starting risk (the "lower than what" part), the message really tells you nothing.

Does the risk reduction information reasonably apply to me?   Learn whether the health message is based on studies of people like you (people of your age and sex and people whose health is like yours). The more you are like the participants in the studies, the more likely you are to face the same starting risk and experience the same benefit.

What are the downsides that come with the risk reduction?   Understand the downsides of the intervention, and decide how much they matter to you. Does the intervention have any life-threatening side effects? What are the important symptom side effects? Don't forget to consider the inconvenience (time, effort, and hassle) and the cost of the intervention to you.

Is the risk reduction—the benefit—worth the downsides?   Look at the benefits and downsides side by side. The more compelling the benefit is—a big change in an outcome you really care about—the more downsides you might be willing to tolerate. But a small change in a surrogate outcome may not be worth even a small sacrifice.

What kind of science is behind the numbers, and who is behind the numbers? Give the most serious consideration to the findings of large, publicly funded, long-term randomized trials that measure an important patient outcome and whose results are published in a peer-reviewed medical journal.

Be very skeptical of the findings of small, industry-funded, uncontrolled, or observational studies that measure surrogate outcomes and whose preliminary results are presented at the meeting of a medical or scientific association. You should also be very skeptical of short-term randomized trials (like many studies of new drugs, which are conducted for only 6 months or less); they may not include enough participants or have a long enough duration to pick up important life-threatening side effects or even to determine the long-term benefit.

GLOSSARY

Absolute risk	The chance that something will happen. Synonyms include *chance*, *probability*, and *risk*. For example, a complete absolute risk statement might read:
	A typical 50-year-old American woman has a 4 in 1,000 chance of dying from breast cancer in the next 10 years.
Absolute risk reduction	An absolute comparison of risks: it tells you how much lower the modified risk is than the starting risk in absolute terms.
	Absolute risk reduction = starting risk − modified risk
	For example, in a randomized trial, women take drug X or a placebo. After 10 years:
	3 out of 1,000 women in the placebo group die of breast cancer (starting risk).
	2 out of 1,000 women in the drug X group die of breast cancer (modifed risk).
	Absolute risk reduction = risk of breast cancer death (placebo group) − risk of breast cancer death (drug X group) = 0.003 − 0.002 = 0.001 = 0.1%
	Here are two ways to express this absolute risk reduction:
	Drug X lowers the 10-year risk of breast cancer death by 0.1 percentage points.
	For every 1,000 women who take drug X for 10 years (instead of a placebo), there will be 1 less breast cancer death.
"Apply to you" (as in "does this risk apply to you?")	Risk information should be derived from studies of people like you. The more similar you are to the people on whom the statistics are based, the more confident you can be that the statistics apply to you. Ideally, this means that the participants in a study were at least people of your age and sex and, preferably, were people whose health is very similar to yours—that is, they have the same diseases you do, or they are healthy like you.

Case-control study	An observational controlled research study in which scientists compare two groups of people, one with a disease or condition and the other without it. The scientists then analyze the two groups to look for clues that would explain the difference (diet, lifestyle, or medical history, for instance). If one group has heart disease and the other does not, for example, the researchers might ask about behaviors such as drinking coffee. If the people with heart disease are more likely to drink coffee, this suggests that coffee may have something to do with heart disease. Because the people in the two groups might differ in many other ways, however, you need to be cautious in interpreting the results. The hypothetical study we just described shows that coffee drinking is associated with heart disease, but it does not prove that coffee drinking causes heart disease.
Chance	The likelihood that something will happen. Synonyms include *absolute risk*, *risk*, and *probability*. In health statistics, chance is referred to as an absolute risk, and a complete statement would include the outcome and the time frame.
Cohort study	A research study in which scientists compare groups of people who differ in some important way. For example, people in one group may drink a lot of coffee, while people in the other group don't drink any. The scientists then observe what happens to the people in each group over time. For example, they might measure what proportion of each group dies from heart disease. Since people in such cohorts can differ in many ways, you need to be cautious in interpreting the results. In this example, people who drink coffee may have other behaviors (such as smoking) that affect their chance of dying from heart disease. This kind of study might show that coffee is associated with heart disease, but it does not prove that coffee causes heart disease.

Control group	In a study, the control group (also called the comparison group) does not receive the therapy being studied (a test or a treatment, for example). The control group typically receives a placebo or conventional medical care, while the intervention group receives the new therapy. Investigators compare the outcomes for the two groups to determine whether the new therapy is better or worse than the current approach.
Death rate	The rate of death in a group or population (also called the mortality rate); often calculated for a specific illness. For example, the 1-year death rate for lung cancer is the number of people in a group who died of lung cancer over the past year divided by the total number of people in the group at the start of the year.
Denominator	The bottom number in a fraction. For example, in the following fraction, 250 is the denominator: $\dfrac{10}{250}$
Downsides	The bad things that can happen if you take an action, including the side effects of drugs or treatments, the inconvenience, and the costs.
Framing	The perspective in which information is presented. Different emotional responses are elicited when the same information is cast in a positive light and in a negative light. For example, the following messages give the same information, but many people find the first message scarier: 9 out of 1,000 fifty-year-old men will die of cancer in the next 10 years. 991 out of 1,000 fifty-year-old men will not die of cancer in the next 10 years.
Modified risk	Your chance of experiencing some outcome *with* an intervention. In a randomized trial, the modified risk is the chance that someone in the intervention group experiences the outcome.

Numerator	The top number in a fraction. For example, in the following fraction, 10 is the numerator: $\dfrac{10}{250}$
Outcome	The event under consideration. Outcomes can include death, both death from all causes combined and death from a specific cause, such as breast cancer or a heart attack (referred to as disease-specific mortality). Types of outcomes include those that people experience directly (patient outcomes), such as needing an operation or being hospitalized, as well as those that are measured in blood tests or X-rays (surrogate outcomes).
Perspective	Comparative information that can help you make a judgment about the magnitude of a risk. For example, knowing that at age 65 a woman who has never smoked has a 5 in 1,000 chance of dying from lung cancer in the next 10 years is much more meaningful if you know how that risk compares to other risks (a 25 in 1,000 chance of dying from a heart attack, a 3 in 1,000 chance of accidental death).
Placebo	An inert substance, sometimes called a "sugar pill" (although it isn't necessarily made from sugar). Placebos are often used in randomized trials to test an intervention. For example, if researchers want to test whether drug X reduces the risk of catching a cold, they can randomly assign participants to either a group who will take drug X or a group who will take an identical-looking but ineffective placebo. At the end of the study, the researchers compare how often people in the two groups caught colds. The purpose of a placebo is to help ensure that patients in each study group are treated in exactly the same way. Without a placebo group, everyone would know which patients were getting the drug under investigation. Those patients might be treated differently—or might report their information differently—and this could bias the results.

Randomized trial	An experiment in which study participants are assigned to study groups solely on the basis of chance—essentially by flipping a coin. This method is the best way to ensure that participants in one group are very similar to those in the other group. The findings from randomized trials are the results that doctors (and you) should trust the most.
Relative risk reduction	A relative comparison of risks: it tells you how much lower the modified risk is relative to the starting risk.

$$\text{Relative risk reduction} = \frac{\text{starting risk} - \text{modified risk}}{\text{starting risk}}$$

$$= \frac{\text{risk of breast cancer death (placebo group)} - \text{risk of breast cancer death (drug X group)}}{\text{risk of breast cancer death (placebo group)}}$$

$$= \frac{3 \text{ out of 1,000 (placebo group)} - 2 \text{ out of 1,000 (drug X group)}}{3 \text{ out of 1,000 (placebo group)}}$$

$$= \frac{.003 - .002}{.003}$$

$$= .33 = 33\% \text{ lower}$$

Here's a way to express this relative risk reduction:

Drug X lowers the 10-year risk of dying from breast cancer by 33 percent.

Risk	The chance that something (good or bad) will happen. Synonyms include *absolute risk*, *chance*, and *probability*.
Screening	Screening means testing people who have no symptoms of a disease to look for hidden, early evidence of the disease. Many tests can be used for screening, including mammography for breast cancer, colonoscopy for colon cancer, and PSA testing for prostate cancer.
	How a test is used determines whether it is a screening test. When a woman with no signs or symptoms of breast cancer gets an annual mammogram, she is getting a screening test. But

when a woman feels a lump in her breast and gets a mammogram, she is getting a diagnostic test in response to a symptom, not a screening test.

Starting risk	Your chance of experiencing some outcome *without* an intervention. In a randomized trial, the starting risk is the chance that someone in the control (or placebo) group experiences the outcome.
Statistics	Statistics are numbers that summarize observations about groups of people. For example, they might summarize typical age or weight by taking the average among a group of people. In this book, statistics summarize the probability of different outcomes by looking at the experience of groups of people. Statistics are useful in predicting what is likely to happen in the future. Most of the numbers in this book are statistics.
Survival rate	The proportion of patients diagnosed with a disease who are alive at some fixed time (typically 5 or 10 years) after diagnosis. Although this statistic can tell you your prognosis and is a good outcome measure of how well treatments work in a randomized trial, it is misleading as a measure of how well screening works. Survival rates will increase whenever cancers are diagnosed earlier, even if the time of death is not postponed.

NUMBER CONVERTER AND RISK CHARTS

Number Converter

1 in __	Decimal	Percent	__ out of 1,000
1 in 1	1.00	100%	1,000 out of 1,000
1 in 2	0.50	50%	500 out of 1,000
1 in 3	0.33	33%	333 out of 1,000
1 in 4	0.25	25%	250 out of 1,000
1 in 5	0.20	20%	200 out of 1,000
1 in 6	0.17	17%	167 out of 1,000
1 in 7	0.14	14%	143 out of 1,000
1 in 8	0.13	13%	125 out of 1,000
1 in 9	0.11	11%	111 out of 1,000
1 in 10	0.10	10%	100 out of 1,000
1 in 20	0.05	5.0%	50 out of 1,000
1 in 25	0.04	4.0%	40 out of 1,000
1 in 50	0.02	2.0%	20 out of 1,000
1 in 100	0.01	1.0%	10 out of 1,000
1 in 200	0.0050	0.50%	5 out of 1,000
1 in 250	0.0040	0.40%	4 out of 1,000
1 in 300	0.0033	0.33%	3.3 out of 1,000
1 in 400	0.0025	0.25%	2.5 out of 1,000
1 in 500	0.0020	0.20%	2.0 out of 1,000
1 in 600	0.0017	0.17%	1.7 out of 1,000
1 in 700	0.0014	0.14%	1.4 out of 1,000

Number Converter *(continued)*

1 in __	Decimal	Percent	__ out of 1,000
1 in 800	0.0013	0.13%	1.3 out of 1,000
1 in 900	0.0011	0.11%	1.1 out of 1,000
1 in 1,000	0.0010	0.10%	1.0 out of 1,000
1 in 2,000	0.00050	0.050%	0.50 out of 1,000
1 in 3,000	0.00033	0.033%	0.33 out of 1,000
1 in 4,000	0.00025	0.025%	0.25 out of 1,000
1 in 5,000	0.00020	0.020%	0.20 out of 1,000
1 in 10,000	0.00010	0.010%	0.10 out of 1,000
1 in 25,000	0.00004	0.004%	0.040 out of 1,000
1 in 50,000	0.00002	0.002%	0.020 out of 1,000
1 in 100,000	0.00001	0.001%	0.010 out of 1,000
1 in 1,000,000	0.000001	0.0001%	0.001 out of 1,000

Note: For numbers less than 1 out of 1,000 (such as 0.50 out of 1,000), it is clearer to recast them as "___ out of 10,000" ("5 out of 10,000," for instance), because it allows you to use a whole number rather than a decimal.

Risk Chart for Men

Find the line closest to your age and smoking status. The numbers in that row tell you how many out of 1,000 men in that group will die in the next 10 years from . . .

Age	Smoking Status	Vascular Disease		Cancer			Infection			Lung Disease	Accidents	All Causes Combined
		Heart Attack	Stroke	Lung	Colon	Prostate	Pneumonia	Flu	AIDS	COPD		
35	Never smoked	1	1						2		5	15
	Smoker	**7**	**1**	**1**					**2**		**5**	**42**
40	Never smoked	3	1	1	1				2		6	24
	Smoker	**14**	**2**	**4**	**1**				**2**	**1**	**6**	**62**
45	Never smoked	6	1	1	1		1		2		6	35
	Smoker	**21**	**3**	**8**	**1**		**1**		**2**	**2**	**6**	**91**
50	Never smoked	11	1	1	2	1	1		1		5	49
	Smoker	**29**	**5**	**18**	**2**	**1**	**1**		**1**	**3**	**5**	**128**
55	Never smoked	19	3	1	3	2	1		1	1	5	74
	Smoker	**41**	**7**	**34**	**3**	**1**	**2**		**1**	**7**	**4**	**178**
60	Never smoked	32	5	2	5	3	2		1	1	5	115
	Smoker	**56**	**11**	**59**	**5**	**3**	**3**		**1**	**16**	**4**	**256**
65	Never smoked	52	9	4	8	6	3			3	6	176
	Smoker	**74**	**16**	**89**	**7**	**6**	**5**			**26**	**5**	**365**
70	Never smoked	87	18	6	10	12	6			5	7	291
	Smoker	**100**	**26**	**113**	**9**	**10**	**9**			**45**	**6**	**511**
75	Never smoked	137	32	8	13	19	12			6	11	449
	Smoker	**140**	**39**	**109**	**11**	**15**	**16**			**60**	**9**	**667**

Source: Steven Woloshin, Lisa Schwartz, and H. Gilbert Welch, "The Risk of Death by Age, Sex, and Smoking Status in the United States: Putting Health Risks in Context," *Journal of the National Cancer Institute* 100 (2008): 845–853.

Note: Shaded portions mean that the chance is less than 1 out of 1,000. People who have never smoked are defined as those who do not smoke now and who have smoked fewer than 100 cigarettes in their lifetime. Smokers are defined as people who have smoked at least 100 cigarettes in their lifetime and who currently smoke (any amount). COPD is chronic obstructive pulmonary disease, which includes emphysema and chronic bronchitis. The numbers in the All Causes Combined column do not represent row totals because they include many other causes of death in addition to the ones listed in the chart.

Risk Chart for Women

Find the line closest to your age and smoking status. The numbers in that row tell you how many out of 1,000 women in that group will die in the next 10 years from . . .

Age	Smoking Status	Vascular Disease		Cancer					Infection			Lung Disease	Accidents	All Causes Combined
		Heart Attack	Stroke	Lung	Breast	Colon	Ovarian	Cervical	Pneumonia	Flu	AIDS	COPD		
35	Never smoked	1			1						1		2	14
	Smoker	**1**	**1**	**1**	**1**						**1**		**2**	**14**
40	Never smoked	1			2	1					1		2	19
	Smoker	**4**	**2**	**4**	**2**						**1**	**1**	**2**	**27**
45	Never smoked	2	1	1	3	1	1				1		2	25
	Smoker	**9**	**3**	**7**	**3**	**1**	**1**				**1**	**2**	**2**	**45**
50	Never smoked	4	1	1	4	1	1		1				2	37
	Smoker	**13**	**5**	**14**	**4**	**1**	**1**		**1**			**4**	**2**	**69**
55	Never smoked	8	2	2	6	2	2	1	1			1	2	55
	Smoker	**20**	**6**	**26**	**5**	**2**	**2**	**1**	**1**			**9**	**2**	**110**
60	Never smoked	14	4	3	7	3	3	1	1			2	2	84
	Smoker	**31**	**8**	**41**	**6**	**3**	**3**	**1**	**2**			**18**	**2**	**167**
65	Never smoked	25	7	5	8	5	4	1	2			3	3	131
	Smoker	**45**	**15**	**55**	**7**	**5**	**3**	**1**	**4**			**31**	**3**	**241**
70	Never smoked	46	14	7	9	7	4	1	4			5	4	207
	Smoker	**66**	**25**	**61**	**8**	**6**	**4**	**1**	**7**			**44**	**4**	**335**
75	Never smoked	86	30	7	10	10	5	1	8			6	7	335
	Smoker	**99**	**34**	**58**	**10**	**9**	**4**		**14**			**61**	**7**	**463**

Source: Steven Woloshin, Lisa Schwartz, and H. Gilbert Welch, "The Risk of Death by Age, Sex, and Smoking Status in the United States: Putting Health Risks in Context," *Journal of the National Cancer Institute* 100 (2008): 845–853.

Note: Shaded portions mean that the chance is less than 1 out of 1,000. People who have never smoked are defined as those who do not smoke now and who have smoked fewer than 100 cigarettes in their lifetime. Smokers are defined as people who have smoked at least 100 cigarettes in their lifetime and who currently smoke (any amount). COPD is chronic obstructive pulmonary disease, which includes emphysema and chronic bronchitis. The numbers in the All Causes Combined column do not represent row totals because they include many other causes of death in addition to the ones listed in the chart.

CREDIBLE SOURCES OF HEALTH STATISTICS

Sources Created Primarily for Consumers

BMJ *(British Medical Journal)* Best Treatments
http://besttreatments.bmj.com/btuk/home.jsp

Medical publishing division of the British Medical Association (no commercial ads allowed). Rates the science supporting the use of operations, tests, and treatments for a variety of conditions. In the United States and Canada, available only with a *Consumer Reports* subscription.

Center for Medical Consumers
www.medicalconsumers.org

Independent, nonprofit organization. Offers a skeptical take on health claims and recent health news. Free.

Consumer Reports Best Buy Drugs*
www.consumerreports.org/health/bestbuy-drugs.htm

Independent, nonprofit organization. Compares the benefits, side effects, and costs of different prescription drugs for the same problem, based on information from the Drug Effectiveness Review Project (see listing on page 131). Free.

Foundation for Informed Medical Decision Making*
www.informedmedicaldecisions.org

Independent, nonprofit organization. Offers decision aids that describe the treatment options and outcomes for various conditions in order to promote patient involvement in decision making. DVDs must be purchased at www.healthdialog.com/hd/Core/CollaborativeCare/videolibrary.htm.

---

* Two of us (Drs. Schwartz and Woloshin) are on the advisory board for Consumer Reports Best Buy Drugs *(unpaid positions). We have been paid consultants reviewing materials for the* Foundation for Informed Medical Decision Making.

Informed Health Online

www.informedhealthonline.org

Institute for Quality and Efficiency in Health Care, an independent, nonprofit organization established by German health care reform legislation. Describes the science supporting the use of operations, tests, and treatments for a variety of conditions. Free.

Ottawa Health Research Institute Patient Decision Aids

http://decisionaid.ohri.ca

Academic affiliate of the University of Ottawa. Provides a comprehensive inventory of decision aids (plus a rating of their quality), and tells patients how to get them. Some are free.

Sources Created Primarily for Physicians and Policy Makers

Agency for Healthcare Research and Quality (AHRQ)

www.ahrq.gov/clinic/epcix.htm

U.S. federal agency under the Department of Health and Human Services. Summarizes all the available data about treatments for specific conditions (look for EPC Evidence Reports). Free.

Cochrane Library

www3.interscience.wiley.com/cgi-bin/mrwhome/106568753/HOME

International, independent, nonprofit organization of researchers. Summarizes all the available data about treatments for specific conditions (look for Cochrane Reviews). Abstracts free, full reports by subscription.

Drug Effectiveness Review Project (DERP)

www.ohsu.edu/drugeffectiveness/reports/final.cfm

Collaboration of public and private organizations developed by Oregon Health and Science University. Provides comparative data on the benefit, side effects, and costs of different prescription drugs for the same problem (source for *Consumer Reports* Best Buy Drugs). Free.

National Institute for Health and Clinical Excellence (NICE)

www.nice.org.uk/guidance/index.jsp?action=byTopic

Independent, nonprofit British organization that advises the British National Health Service. Summarizes all the available data about treatments for specific conditions (look for NICE Guidance). Free.

Physician Data Query (PDQ)—National Cancer Institute

www.cancer.gov/cancertopics/pdq

U.S. federal government (part of the National Cancer Institute). Summarizes all the available data about cancer prognosis and treatments (look for Cancer Information Summaries). Free.

U.S. Food and Drug Administration (FDA), Center for Drug Evaluation and Research

www.fda.gov/cder/index.html

U.S. federal agency under the Department of Health and Human Services, which reviews and approves new and generic drugs. To look up individual drugs, go to www.accessdata.fda.gov/scripts/cder/drugsatfda/index.cfm. After you choose a drug from the index, the Drug Details page appears. If you click Approval History, you may be able to access a Review and then a Medical Review. The Medical Review contains all the relevant randomized trials submitted to the FDA for approval. From the Drug Details page, you can also access Label Information, when it is available (the package insert that comes with prescription drugs and summarizes excerpts of the review documents). *Warning:* This site can be challenging. The review documents can be hundreds of pages, and there may be multiple entries for the same drug (because it is used for multiple purposes). Free.

US Preventive Services Task Force

www.ahrq.gov/clinic/uspstfix.htm

Independent panel of experts sponsored by AHRQ. Summarizes the available data about preventive services. After you choose a topic, you'll see the relevant recommendations; at the bottom of the list, you can click Best-Evidence Systematic Review under Supporting Documents. Free.

Chapter 2. Putting Risk in Perspective

1. Steven Woloshin, Lisa Schwartz, and H. Gilbert Welch, "Risk Charts: Putting Cancer in Context," *Journal of the National Cancer Institute* 94 (2002): 799–804, available at http://jnci.oxfordjournals.org/cgi/reprint/94/11/799.

2. Steven Woloshin, Lisa Schwartz, and H. Gilbert Welch, "The Risk of Death by Age, Sex, and Smoking Status in the United States: Putting Health Risks in Context," *Journal of the National Cancer Institute* 100 (2008): 845–853, available at www.vaoutcomes.org/books.php.

Chapter 4. Judging the Benefit of a Health Intervention

1. T. R. Pederson, "Randomised Trial of Cholesterol Lowering in 4444 Patients with Coronary Heart Disease: The Scandinavian Simvastatin Survival Study (4S)," *Lancet* 344 (1994): 1383–1389.

2. You may be wondering why the risk of heart attack death in the placebo group in the Zocor study, which included people age 35 to 70, is so high: 8.5% (85 per 1,000 people) over 5 years. According to the risk charts, the *10 year* risk of heart disease death doesn't reach that level for men until age 70, and for women until age 75. The explanation is simple. The risk charts show the average risk for people at each age. But the people in the Zocor study were not "average." They all were high risk for heart disease death because they had already had one prior heart attack. This highlights the importance of knowing whom health statistics are based on: characteristics like age, gender, and, in this case, health conditions powerfully influence risk.

3. Lisa Schwartz, Steven Woloshin, Evan Dvorin, and H. Gilbert Welch, "Ratio Measures in Leading Medical Journals: Structured Review of Accessibility of Underlying Absolute Risks," *British Medical Journal* 333 (2006): 1248–1250, available at www.vaoutcomes.org/books.php.

4. Steven Woloshin and Lisa Schwartz, "Press Releases: Translating Research into News," *Journal of the American Medical Association* 287 (2002): 2856–2858, available at www.vaoutcomes.org/books.php.

5. Steven Woloshin and Lisa Schwartz, "Media Reporting on Scientific Meeting Presentations: More Caution Needed," *Medical Journal of Australia* 184 (2006): 576–580, available at https://www.mja.com.au/public/issues/184_11_050606/wol10024_fm.pdf; Lisa Schwartz and Steven Woloshin, "News Media Coverage of Screening Mammography for Women in Their 40s and Tamoxifen for Primary Prevention of Breast Cancer," *Journal of the American Medical Association* 287 (2002): 3136–3142, available at www.vaoutcomes.org/books.php; Ray Moynihan, Lisa Bero, Dennis Ross-Degnan, David Henry, Kirby Lee, Judy Watkins, Connie Mah, and Stephen Soumerai, "Coverage by the Media of the Benefits and Risks of Medications," *New England Journal of Medicine* 342 (2000): 1645–1650; Alan Cassels, Merrilee Hughes, Carol Cole, Barbara Mintzes, Joel Lexchin, and James McCormack, "Drugs in the News: An Analysis of Canadian Newspaper Coverage of New Prescription Drugs," *Canadian Medical Journal* 168 (2003): 1133–1137.

6. Steven Woloshin, Lisa Schwartz, Jennifer Tremmel, and H. Gilbert Welch, "Direct to Consumer Drug Advertisements: What Are Americans Being Sold?" *Lancet* 358 (2001): 1141–1146, available at www.vaoutcomes.org/books.php; Robert Bell, Michael Wilkes, and Richard Kravitz, "The Educational Value of Consumer-Targeted Prescription Drug Advertising," *Journal of Family Practice* 49 (2000): 1092–1098.

Chapter 5. Not All Benefits Are Equal

1. Writing Group for the Women's Health Initiative Investigators, "Risks and Benefits of Estrogen plus Progestin in Healthy Postmenopausal Women: Principal Results from the Women's Health Initiative Randomized Controlled Trial," *Journal of the American Medical Association* 288 (2002): 321–333.

2. Richard Bogan, June Fry, Markus Schmidt, Stanley Carson, and Sally Ritchie for the TREAT RLS US (Therapy with Ropinirole Efficacy and Tolerability in RLS US) Study Group, *Mayo Clinic Proceedings* 81 (2006): 17–27.

Chapter 6. Consider the Downsides

1. Andrew Krystal, James Walsh, Eugene Laska, Judy Caron, David Amato, Thomas Wessel, and Thomas Roth, "Sustained Efficacy of Eszopiclone over 6 Months of Nightly Treatment: Results of a Randomized, Double-Blind, Placebo-Controlled Study in Adults with Chronic Insomnia," *Sleep* 26 (2003): 793–799.

2. Table data taken from Krystal et al., "Sustained Efficacy of Eszopiclone."

3. Bernard Fisher, Joseph P. Costantino, D. Lawrence Wickerham, Carol K.

Redmond, Maureen Kavanah, Walter M. Cronin, Victor Vogel, André Robidoux, Nikolay Dimitrov, James Atkins, Mary Daly, Samuel Wieand, Elizabeth Tan-Chiu, Leslie Ford, Norman Wolmark, and other National Surgical Adjuvant Breast and Bowel Project investigators, "Tamoxifen for Prevention of Breast Cancer: Report of the National Surgical Adjuvant Breast and Bowel Project P-1 Study," *Journal of the National Cancer Institute* 90 (1998): 1371–1388.

Chapter 7. Do the Benefits Outweigh the Downsides?

1. Andrew Krystal, James Walsh, Eugene Laska, Judy Caron, David Amato, Thomas Wessel, and Thomas Roth, "Sustained Efficacy of Eszopiclone over 6 Months of Nightly Treatment: Results of a Randomized, Double-Blind, Placebo-Controlled Study in Adults with Chronic Insomnia," *Sleep* 26 (2003): 793–799.

2. Bernard Fisher, Joseph P. Costantino, D. Lawrence Wickerham, Carol K. Redmond, Maureen Kavanah, Walter M. Cronin, Victor Vogel, André Robidoux, Nikolay Dimitrov, James Atkins, Mary Daly, Samuel Wieand, Elizabeth Tan-Chiu, Leslie Ford, Norman Wolmark, and other National Surgical Adjuvant Breast and Bowel Project investigators, "Tamoxifen for Prevention of Breast Cancer: Report of the National Surgical Adjuvant Breast and Bowel Project P-1 Study," *Journal of the National Cancer Institute* 90 (1998): 1371–1388. In the table shown in the chapter 7 text, 5-year risks were calculated from the annual rates presented in this article.

Chapter 8. Beware of Exaggerated Importance

1. Thomas Maugh, "Study Calls for Routine CT Scans for Smokers; Imaging Can Detect Lung Cancer Early, Boosting Survival Rates. But Some Experts Say More Research Is Needed," *Los Angeles Times,* October 26, 2006, A18.

2. Pamela Marcus, Erik Bergstralh, Richard Fagerstrom, David Williams, Robert Fontana, William Taylor, and Phillip Prorok, "Lung Cancer Mortality in the Mayo Lung Project: Impact of Extended Follow-Up," *Journal of the National Cancer Institute* 92 (2000): 1308–1316.

3. H. Gilbert Welch, Lisa Schwartz, and Steven Woloshin, "Are Increasing 5-Year Survival Rates Evidence of Progress against Cancer?" *Journal of the American Medical Association* 283 (2000): 2975–2978, available at www.vaoutcomes.org/books.php.

4. L.A.G. Ries, C.L. Kosary, B.F. Hankey, B.A. Miller, L. Clegg, and B.K. Edwards, eds., *SEER Cancer Statistics Review, 1973–1996,* National Cancer Institute, Bethesda, Md., 1999, available at http://seer.cancer.gov/csr/1973_1996/index.html (1950 data available in the Overview document); L.A.G. Ries, D. Melbert, M. Krapcho, D.G. Stinchcomb, N. Howlader, M.J. Horner, A. Mariotto, B.A.

Miller, E. J. Feuer, S. F. Altekruse, D. R. Lewis, L. Clegg, M. P. Eisner, M. Reichman, and B. K. Edwards, eds., *SEER Cancer Statistics Review, 1975–2005,* National Cancer Institute, Bethesda, Md., available at http://seer.cancer.gov/csr/1975_2005/, based on November 2007 SEER data submission, posted to the SEER website, 2008.

5. SEER (Surveillance, Epidemiology, and End Results) stage-specific survival rates (and other cancer statistics) are available at http://seer.cancer.gov/cgi-bin/csr/1975_2004/search.pl.

6. See also H. Gilbert Welch, Steven Woloshin, and Lisa Schwartz, "How Two Studies on Cancer Screening Led to Two Results," *New York Times,* March 13, 2007, F5, F8, available at www.nytimes.com/2007/03/13/health/13lung.html; H. Gilbert Welch, Steven Woloshin, Lisa Schwartz, Leon Gordis, Peter Gotzsche, Russell Harris, Barnett Kramer, and David Ransonhoff, "Overstating the Evidence for Lung Cancer Screening: The I-ELCAP Study," *Archives of Internal Medicine* 167 (2007): 1–7, available at http://archinte.ama-assn.org/cgi/content/full/167/21/2289.

Chapter 9. Beware of Exaggerated Certainty

1. Daniel G. Hackam and Donald Redelmeier, "Translation of Research Evidence from Animals to Humans," *Journal of the American Medical Association* 296 (2006): 1731–1732.

2. Lisa Schwartz, Steven Woloshin, and H. Gilbert Welch, "Can Patients Interpret Health Information? An Assessment of the Medical Data Interpretation Test," *Medical Decision Making* 25 (2005): 290–300, available at www.vaoutcomes.org/books.php.

3. Steven Woloshin, Lisa Schwartz, and H. Gilbert Welch, "The Effectiveness of a Primer to Help People Understand Risk: Two Randomized Trials in Distinct Populations," *Annals of Internal Medicine* 146, no. 4 (2007): 256–265, available at www.annals.org/cgi/content/full/146/4/256.

4. To learn more about research design and the importance of randomized trials, see Imogen Evans, Hazel Thornton, and Iain Chalmers, *Testing Treatments: Better Research for Better Healthcare* (London: British Library, 2006).

5. Lisa Schwartz, Steven Woloshin, and Linda Baczek, "Media Coverage of Scientific Meetings: Too Much, Too Soon?" *Journal of the American Medical Association* 287 (2002): 2859–2863, available at www.vaoutcomes.org/books.php.

6. Karen Lasser, Paul Allen, Steffie Woolhandler, David Himmelstein, Sidney Wolfe, and David Bor, "Timing of New Black Box Warnings and Withdrawals for Prescription Medications," *Journal of the American Medical Association* 287 (2002): 2215–2220.

Chapter 10. Who's Behind the Numbers?

1. Justin Bekelman, Yan Li, and Cary Gross, "Scope and Impact of Financial Conflicts of Interest in Biomedical Research: A Systematic Review," *Journal of the American Medical Association* 289 (2003): 454–465.

2. H. Gilbert Welch and Juliana Mogielnicki, "Presumed Benefit: Lessons from the American Experience with Marrow Transplantation for Breast Cancer," *British Medical Journal* 324 (2002): 1088–1092, available at www.pubmedcentral.nih.gov/articlerender.fcgi?artid=1123033.

3. Lisa Schwartz and Steven Woloshin, "The Case for Letting Information Speak for Itself," *Effective Clinical Practice* 4 (2001): 76–79, available at www.vaoutcomes.org/books.php.

4. The National Library of Medicine's indexes of the medical literature are available at www.ncbi.nlm.nih.gov/PubMed.

5. The federal government's registry of clinical trials (ClinicalTrials.gov) lists federally and privately supported clinical trials conducted in the United States and around the world, and includes details about the study design and funding. It is available at www.clinicaltrials.gov/ct2/search.

6. The Integrity in Science Project tracks more than 200 science-based federal advisory committees for undisclosed conflicts of interest and monitors the media and scientific literature for failure to disclose conflicts. It is available at www.cspinet.org/integrity.

diagnoses *(continued)*
diagnosis and survival statistics, 96
downsides, 67, 118, 122. *See also* side effects
drug ads, 46, 53, 59–60, 87; side effects in, 68. *See also* drug benefits, judging
drug approvals, premature, 106–7
drug benefits, judging, 37–53; calculating risk reductions, 45; clofibrate example, 58; HRT example, 58–59, 103, 106; information sources, 130–32; Lunesta example, 68–72, 75–77; new drugs, 106–7; Nolvadex example, 72–74, 77–81; prescription drug facts boxes, 82; questions to ask, 38–40; relative vs. absolute risk reduction, 40–46; Requip example, 62; surrogate outcomes vs. patient outcomes, 57–60, 63, 88, 118; using a comparison table, 46–47, 82–83; Zocor example, 37–40, 42–45, 50–51. *See also* side effects
Drug Effectiveness Review Project (DERP), 130, 131

estrogen replacement, 58–59, 103, 106

FDA (U.S. Food and Drug Administration), 46, 82; drug approvals and regulation, 68, 70, 106; website for drug research, 132
financial disclosures: health research, 113
flu risk, 128–29
Foundation for Informed Medical Decision Making, 130
fractions, risk expressed as, 13

framing of health messages, 20–21, 27, 44, 110, 112; defined, 122; reframing, 27–28, 34; relative risk reduction, 46

gender-specific risks and outcomes, 14–15, 21–22; risk charts, 128–29

health interventions: credible information sources, 130–32; downsides, 67, 118, 122. *See also* benefit, understanding; drug benefits, judging; risk reduction; screening tests; side effects
health messages, evaluating, 33–34, 87–89; importance of perspective, 21–22, 23–24, 123; questions to ask, 117–19; source and credibility issues, 87–88, 109–13. *See also* framing of health messages
health research, 101–7; definitions, 121, 122, 123, 124; financial disclosures, 113; preliminary findings, 106, 119; questions to ask, 119; randomized trials, 61, 96–97, 103–6, 124, 125; source and credibility issues, 109–13, 119; starting risk omitted from findings, 48, 52–53; study types and believability, 102–6, 119
heart attacks: cholesterol-lowering drugs and, 57, 58; HRT and, 58–59, 103; risk of, 32, 33; risk of death from, 45–46; vitamins and, 59
heart disease: HRT and, 103; risk charts, 128–29
HRT (hormone replacement therapy), 58–59, 103, 106

inconvenience, 67, 122
infection risk, 128–29

Informed Health Online, 131
Integrity in Science Project, 113

Journal of the National Cancer Institute, 24

life-threatening side effects, 67, 72–74, 79, 80–81
lifetime risks, 18–19
Lunesta, 68–72, 75–77
lung cancer risk, 32, 128–29
lung cancer screening, 90–93
lung disease risk, 128–29

March of Dimes, 112
medical interventions. *See* drug benefits, judging; health interventions; side effects
medical journals, 52
melanoma, 95
men: gender-specific risks of death, 14–15, 21–22; risk chart for, 128
modified risk, 41–43, 47, 48, 122; in risk reduction calculations, 45, 48–52

National Cancer Institute Physician Data Query, 132
National Institute for Health and Clinical Excellence (NICE), 131
National Library of Medicine, 113
news reports, 53, 87–88, 110, 111
NICE (National Institute for Health and Clinical Excellence), 132
Nolvadex, 72–74, 77–81
number conversions, 17, 126–27

observational studies, 102–3, 121
Ottawa Health Research Institute, 131
outcomes, 33, 55, 88; death, 56, 62, 63, 64; defined, 123; diag-

tables, to analyze potential benefits and side effects, 46–47, 82–83

tamoxifen. *See* Nolvadex

tests: improved test results as benefit, 55–56, 57, 59–60, 64; screening tests, 90–99, 124

test tube research, 101–2

time frames: in risk analysis, 17–19, 117; in survival statistics, 90, 125

treatments, 6. *See also* health interventions; side effects; *specific drugs*

U.S. Food and Drug Administration. *See* FDA

U.S. Preventive Services Task Force, 132

vascular disease risk, 128–29

vitamins, 59

websites, 130–32

Welch, H. Gilbert, 99

women: gender-specific risks of death, 14–15, 21–22; risk chart examples, 24–28, 29–30; risk chart for, 129

Women's Health Initiative, 58

Zocor, 37–40, 42–45, 50–51

Text:	11.5/15.7 Adobe Garamond Pro
Display:	Officina Sans family
Design and composition:	Barbara Haines
Printer and binder:	Maple-Vail Book Manufacturing Group

Northport-East Northport Public Library

To view your patron record from a computer, click on
the Library's homepage: **www.nenpl.org**

You may:
- request an item be placed on hold
- renew an item that is overdue
- view titles and due dates checked out on your card
- view your own outstanding fines

**151 Laurel Avenue
Northport, NY 11768
631-261-6930**